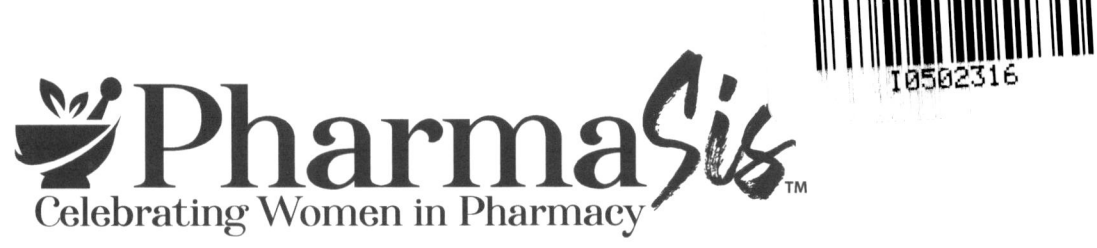

Executive Editor in Chief
Dr. Jerrica Dodd

Creative Director Shannon S. G. Jarrett - Speak Beautiful

Cover Photographer Tessa Swarthout - Tessa Marie Studios

Cover Fashion Stylist Tijuana Faison - Design Faze Boutique

Cover Hair Stylist - Alicia Igess - Urban Tangles Salon

Cover Makeup Artist - Sydney King

PharmaSisMag.com

Copyright © 2024 PharmaSis Magazine

All rights reserved. No part of this book may be reproduced or used in any manner without the prior written permission of the copyright owner, except for the use of brief quotations in a book review.

To request permissions, contact the publisher at
www.pharamasismag.com

Printed by PharmaSis Magazine, in the United States of America.

First printing, 2024.

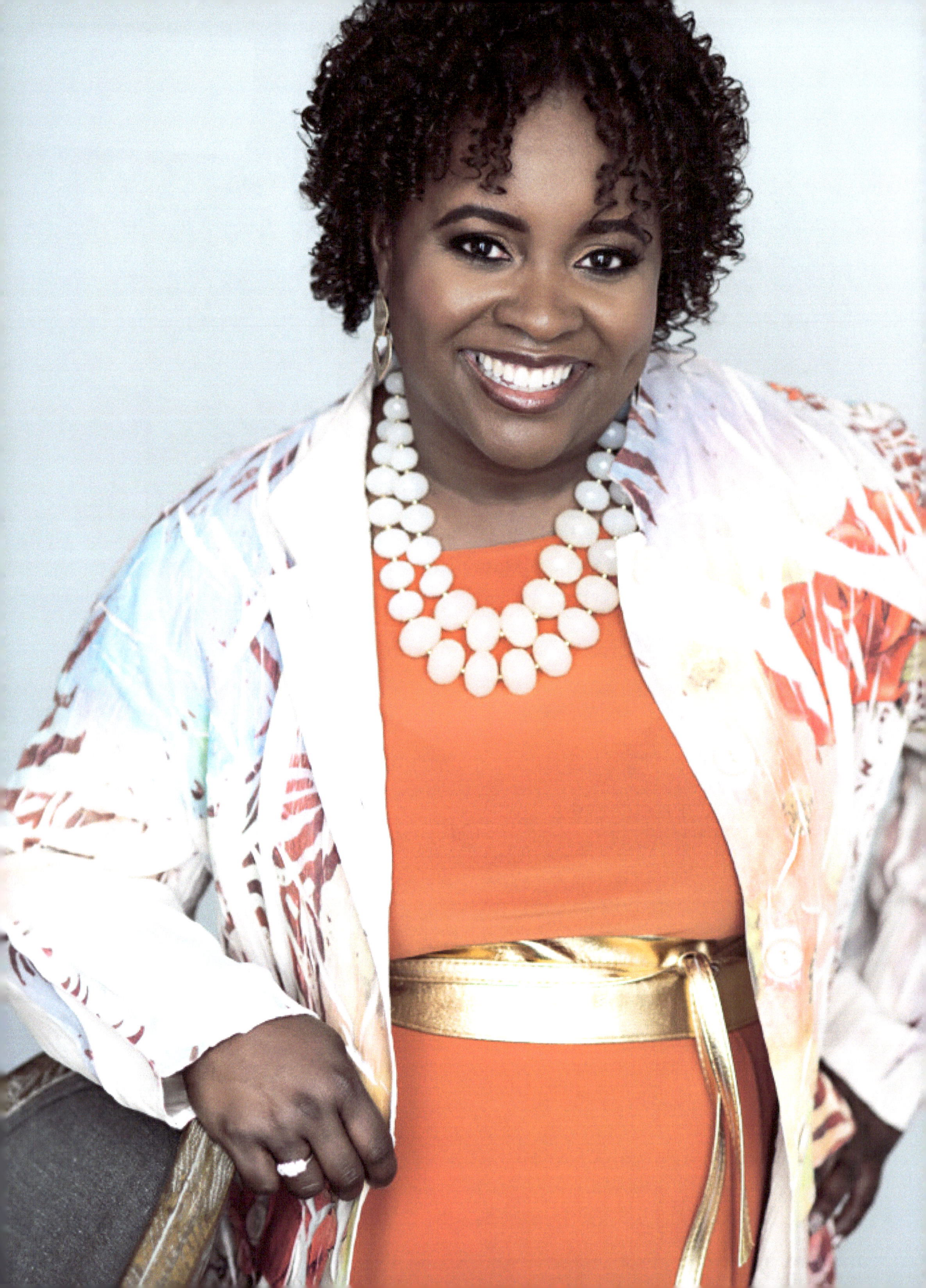

WELCOME TO THE PHARMASIS MAGAZINE

I am so pleased to bring you more of the faces of women in pharmacy who are moving and building their dreams. I want to get you ready for meeting a wonderful group of women who are driven by their convictions and their passions to fill gaps while developing themselves and their world around them. My excitement to feature women in the magazine cannot be paralleled!

Dive in and enjoy! Share this magazine with a woman in pharmacy who may be looking for inspiration, with a student interested in pursuing a STEM career so she can see role models, and finally anyone who is open to learn that "Pharmacists do THAT Too!".

Enjoy the journey!

Jerrica

Dr. Jerrica Dodd
Founder/Editor, PharmaSis Magazine
Founder/CEO, Your Pharmacy Advocate
PharmD, Florida A&M Univ. 1998
MS, Pharmacy Administration, The Ohio State Univ. 2000
MS, Applied Pharmacoeconomics, Univ. of Florida 2012

FROM THE EDITOR

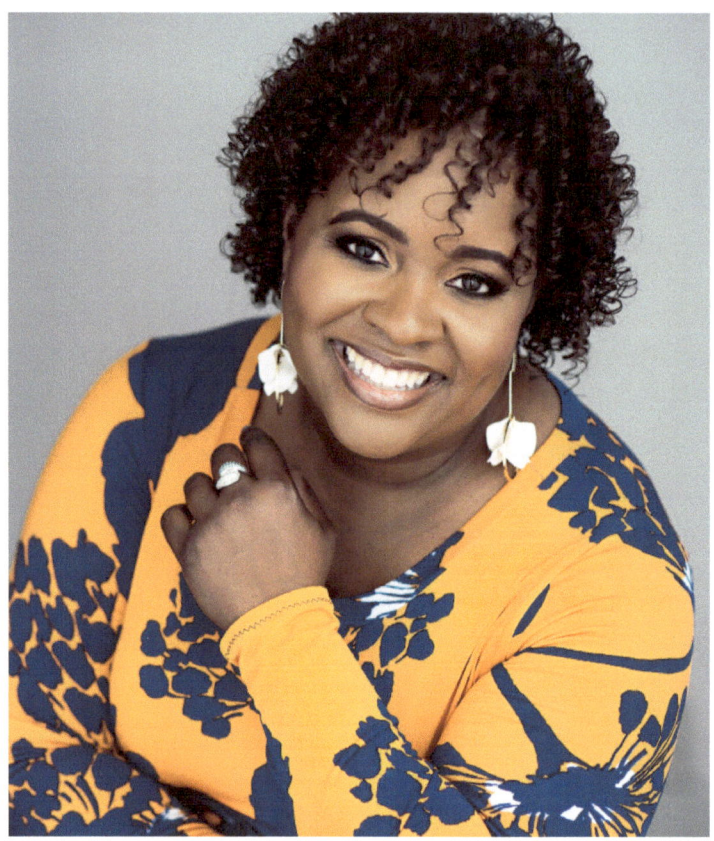

Being the Executive Editor of PharmaSis Magazine is like a dream come true! Through this magazine, I have met so many amazing women in pharmacy and I am in the process of taking this vision around the world to meet even more women in pharmacy! I am thrilled to publish the magazine each time as it never gets old meeting and featuring women building their dreams! Their dreams are URGENT! My dreams are URGENT! Your dreams are URGENT!

Love and hugs,
Jerrica

on the cover

Celebrate Health & Wellness
Dr. Katashia Partee Kendrick
6

Birthing Possibilities
Dr. Katashia Partee Kendrick
13

INSIDE THIS ISSUE

Be Curious, Dream Big
Dr. Myungsun (Sunny) Ro
16

What Breaking the "Glass Ceiling" Means to Me
Dr. Myungsun (Sunny) Ro
23

The Heart and Mind of Style
A Stylish Conversation with Dr. Danielle and Elle Renée
24

Beyond Your Comfort Zone
Dr. Blair Thielemier
28

Learning to Battle Self-Critism
Dr. Janhavi Punyarthi
32

Intentional Style
Elle René
34

Start. Go. Do.
Dr. Leslie Hodge
36

The Art of Making Time
Kristine Cline
40

I Dare You to Bare Your Soles
Dr. Gilda M. Jefferson
42

Author Spotlight
Dr. Gilda M. Jefferson
44

Leading with Compassion
Whitney Jo Hummel
46

A Special Message to Pharmacy Technicians
Whitney Jo Hummel
52

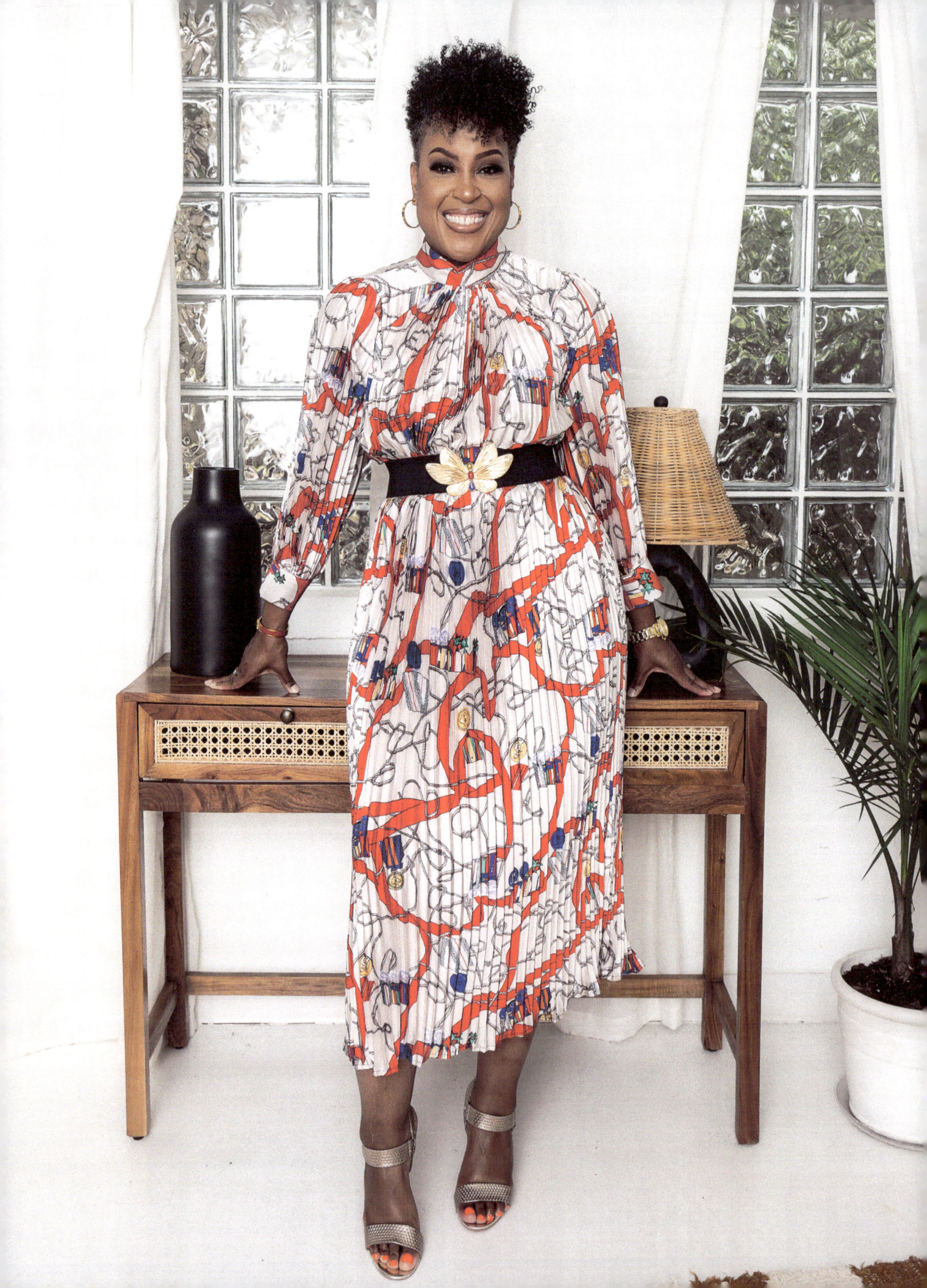

CLINICAL PHARMACY & INTEGRATIVE
HEALTH PRACTITIONER

DR. KATASHIA PARTEE KENDRICK

Celebrate Health & Wellness

HOUSTON, TEXAS | **PHARMACY SCHOOL:** XAVIER UNIVERSITY OF LOUISIANA COLLEGE OF PHARMACY | **DEGREES:** DOCTOR OF PHARMACY | **PREVIOUS CAREER:** CLINICAL PHARMACY PRACTITIONER | **NOW CAREER:** CLINICAL PHARMACY PRACTITIONER & INTEGRATIVE HEALTH PRACTITIONER

Tell your story…how did you get here?

My Story…

Have you ever been broken? Have you ever struggled with fear or grief? What about depression? I was all of those things; utter brokenness. This brokenness ballooned into paralyzing fear. Let me take you back to the beginning. When I was in the 5th grade, I overheard a teacher's assistant say, "I don't like Katashia's voice." My little mind could not comprehend how my voice had somehow moved this grown woman to feel so strongly.

Somehow that singular statement prompted me to dim my light; I became a selective mute. From that day forward, I dreaded having to speak in public. Even when I felt passionate about this or that, I still could not muster the strength to break through the silence because someone who should have been there to encourage me and help mold me into a powerful being had taught me, I was inadequate in some way.

Throughout my formative years, I continued to dim my light well into adulthood. During this time, my sense of self was further challenged as I lost my father, learned of my infertility struggles (endometriosis and fibroids), received a diagnosis of irritable bowel syndrome and the coup de gras was the looming diagnosis of high blood pressure after I found myself weighing over 290 pounds. Due to my own struggles with infertility and IBS, no conventional doctor could truly help me. I had a hysterectomy at the age of 38 due to fibroids and endometriosis. I've never been pregnant. GI doctors told me to take pills daily for my chronic constipation. I refused to live my life like that. I looked into functional medicine and it changed my life. In that moment I had to fight through the fear and find my power. I talked WITH MY CREATOR and he showed me what I needed to do to heal both the physical and psychological wounds I endured. Now my scars tell a story. One of overcoming obesity through understanding gut health and two, finding peace on the other side of my dark, painful infertility journey.

Today I am here having learned how to turn fear into FAITH, grief into GRATEFULNESS and depression into DETERMINATION. I knew I couldn't keep this breakthrough for myself as a singular win. I knew I had to pay it forward. My story might just help someone else find their voice. Today, I have lost over 100 pounds without surgery and off blood pressure medicine. I want to share my journey with others. I found purpose through my pain with infertility and IBS-C. I started Celebrate Health & Wellness Consulting (a virtual practice) using functional medicine lab testing to help women address the root cause of their gut and hormone imbalances. I became a Certified Integrative Health Practitioner (through the Integrative Health Institute) and continue to practice as a Clinical Pharmacy Practitioner in

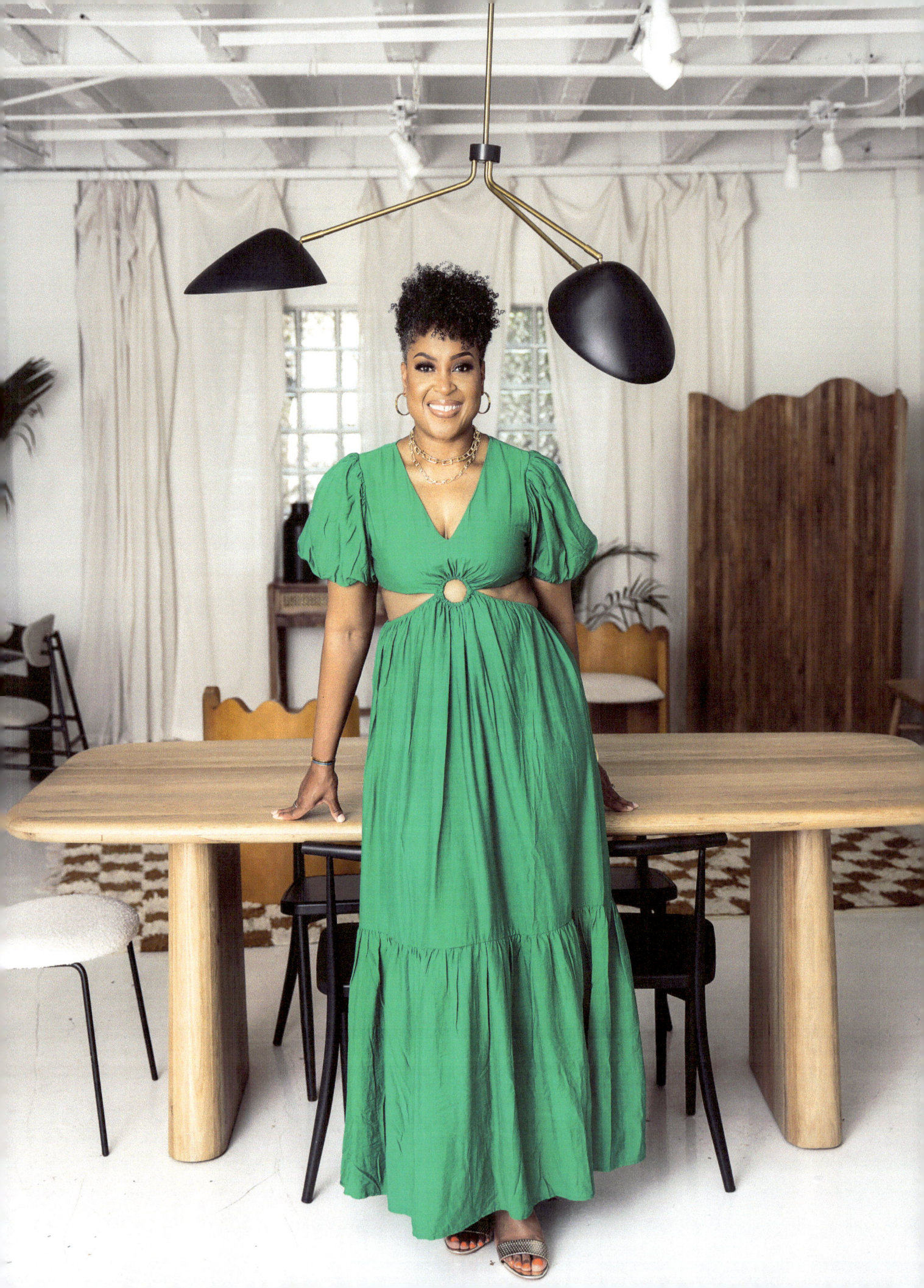

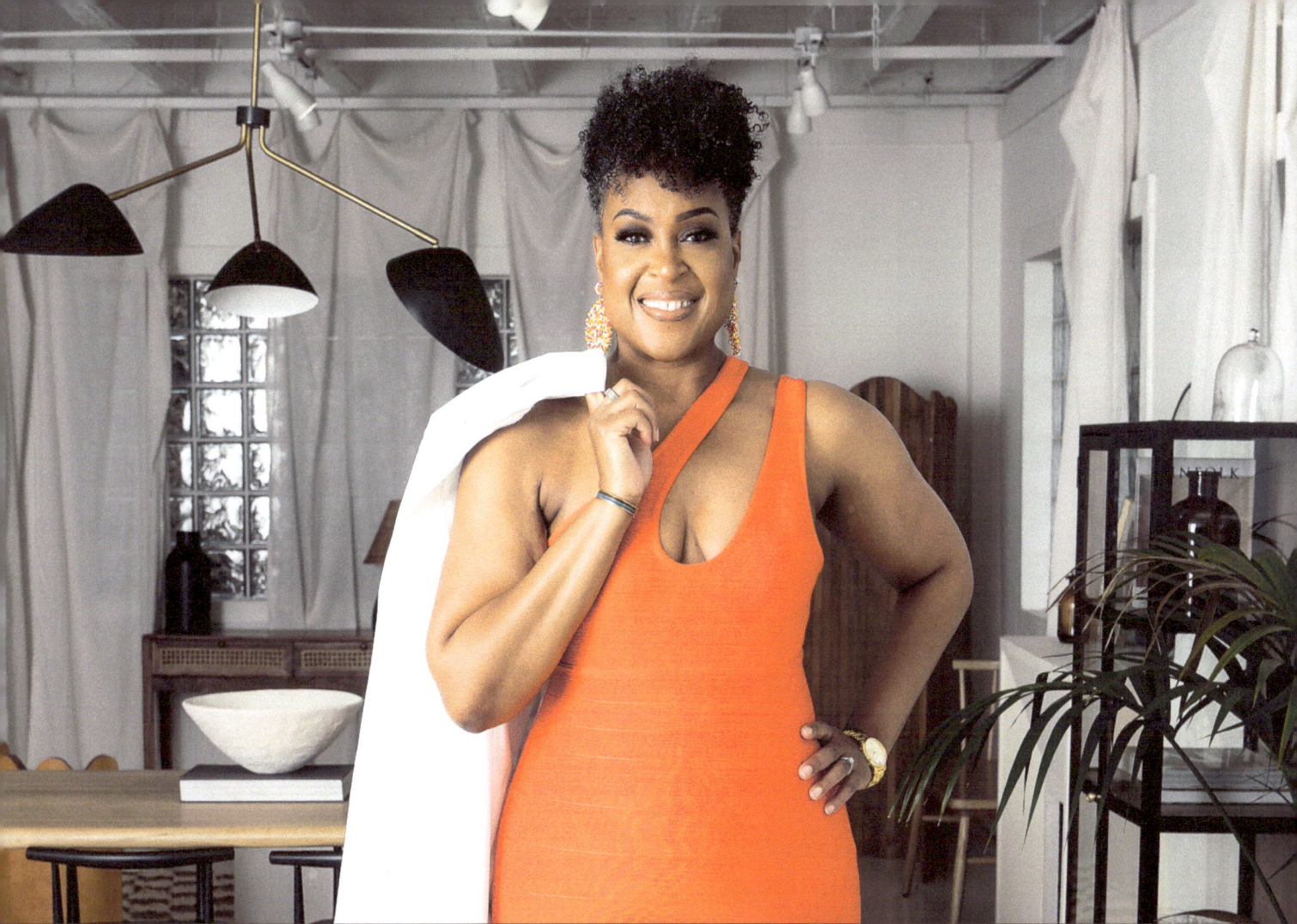

Ambulatory Care. Also, I am an Infertility Survivor & Advocate. Now, I am an Ambassador for Filling Empty Wombs (an organization helping to bring awareness to infertility and provide financial assistance to families seeking alternative way to have a family) and heavily involved with We Can Wear White (an organization bringing awareness to fibroids).

I am Dr. Katashia Partee Kendrick best known as Dr. Katashia or the Gut Health PharmD. I am looking forward to educating so many women about gut health and sharing my infertility journey. I found my voice and my mission is to help other women to find theirs.

Describe what you are building/have built (your business; your career)

I am the Founder and CEO of Celebrate Health & Wellness Consulting, LLC, an online company that provides Integrative Health & Functional Medicine Services and Health & Wellness coaching to busy, professional women. We also offer medication therapy management and CBD consulting. I recently launched my own CBD product line. Celebrate Health & Wellness Consulting, LLC was birth from my own personal health challenges and today I'm living a healthier lifestyle and want to show others how they can possess the freedom I enjoy with better health. I have over 15 years of experience in ambulatory care pharmacy and I am very passionate about anything and everything wellness. I specialize in gut health and chronic disease medication management. Gut health is near and dear to me because of my own struggles with irritable bowel syndrome with constipation. By understanding my food triggers and repairing my gut, I was able to become rebalanced, renewed and rejuvenated through functional medicine lab testing and integrative health strategies and I want other women like me to experience the same breakthrough.

The vision of Celebrate Health & Wellness Consulting, LLC is to educate, inspire, and empower women to live healthier lives and to understand the power of a healthy gut.

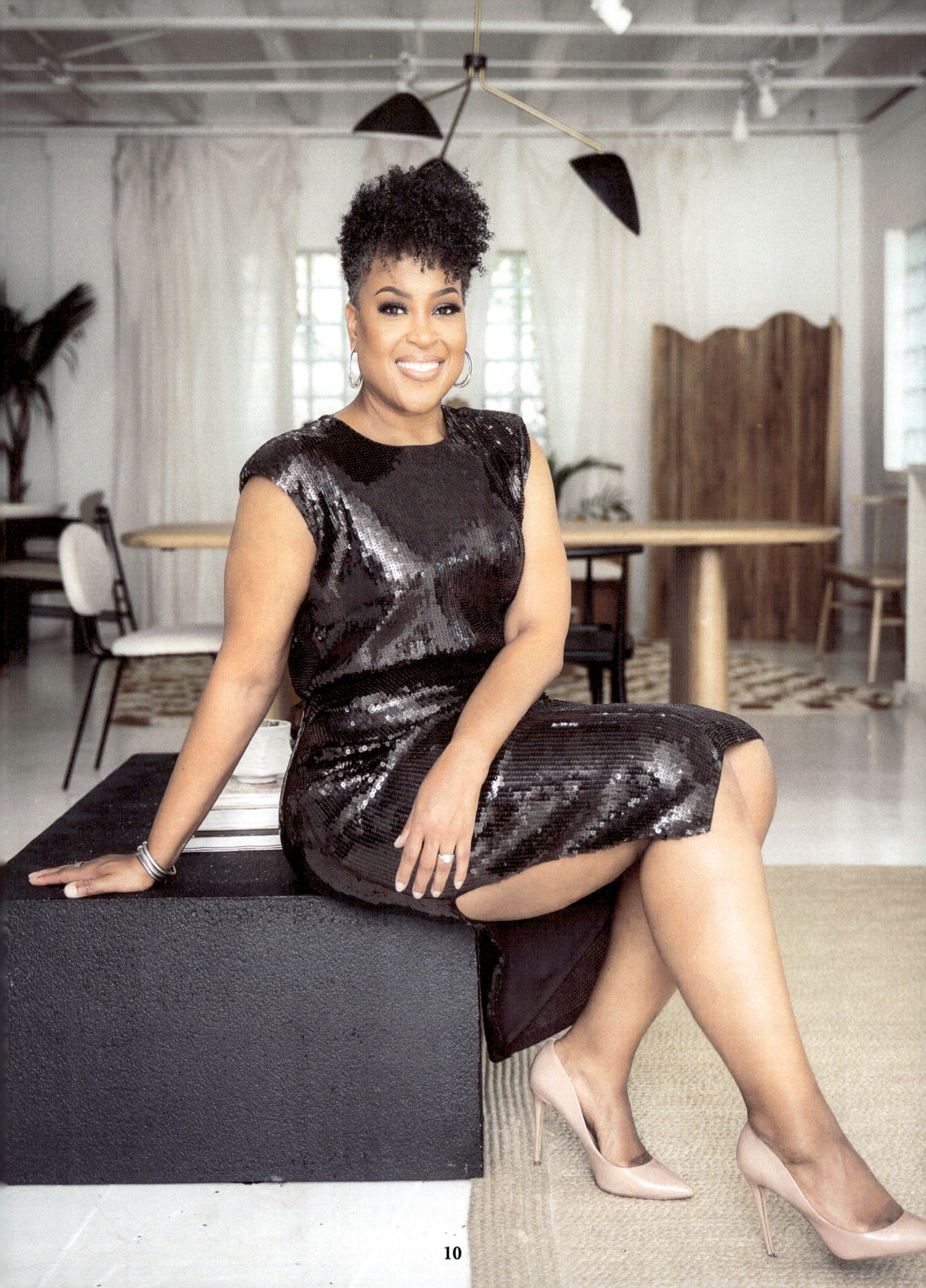

What's been your biggest lesson you have learned along your journey?

The road traveled wasn't easy but it was certainly worth it. Struggles and successes are not new to me, however, choosing to pursue entrepreneurship was absolutely new for me. However, learning from my struggles and failures allowed me to grow personally and professionally, to be patient but persistent and to never give up on my dreams. The lessons I have learned have grown my prayer life for sure. It has allowed me to accept that there will be challenges but I am built for this. The "W" is mine for the taking. I believe people who are successful are those who are resilient. Struggle is a part of life. How we face those challenges and how quickly we bounce back and give ourselves grace is key to growth.

How do you respond to fear?

To be transparent, I have my struggles with fear. However, I truly face those fears now and push through. I don't want my fears to become my limits. Therefore, I have learned to turn fear into FAITH! I decided that I won't let fear decide my future. Take the risk! Why not?

What does it mean to be considered a leader in your profession and industry?

To be considered a leader in your profession and/or industry, one must have a servant's heart. Helping people without expectations. Leadership is about the impact you leave behind while inspiring and empowering along the way.

At this time, pharmacists are being challenged to think out of the box more than ever. What advice do you have for the pharmacist who is wondering how to do that?

Thinking out of the box means doing something that you wouldn't normally do. If you want to start a business, spend time with people who have started a business. If you have an idea, write it down in a notebook and add to it. Let your idea evolve into something that scares you. That's how greatness starts.

Who do you look up to or model yourself after (personal or professional)?

My mother, Minnie P. Partee is who I model myself after and look up to. She laid the foundation for me and it is the blueprint for how I handle life, the good and the bad. My mother is the strongest person I know and has always been there for me. She has taught me life lessons that I will never forget. She is full of wisdom and the way she expresses herself is undeniably like no other. I owe everything to her and I am grateful that God saw fit to make her my mother. I am a strong woman because a strong woman raised me.

What message would you share with other colleagues in pharmacy?

Life is all about risks. It was risky for me to think I could graduate from a 4-year college when no one in my family had accomplished this task. It was risky for me to move to New Orleans to attend pharmacy school knowing the degree of separation anxiety I had previously experienced being away from my family whom I am very close to. It was a risk to start an online health & wellness practice during COVID-19. However, its' been said that without risk, there is no reward. The bottom line is if there's a chance of doing something that will make you happy, risk it and give it your best shot.

What's next for you and/or your business?

For me, I would love to continue to share my infertility journey alongside my husband especially on bigger platforms to reach more people. As well as, possibly start my own non-profit to provide grants to families seeking assistance.

For Celebrate Health & Wellness, continue to help women address the root cause of their gut & hormonal imbalances, expand product line to supplements and other wellness products or future retreats. Right now, I am enjoying the journey while chasing my dreams.

Where can we find you to further connect? (no email addresses or phone numbers please)

Website: drkatashia.com
Instagram: @drkatashia
Facebook: Celebrate Health & Wellness
LinkedIn: Katashia Partee Kendrick

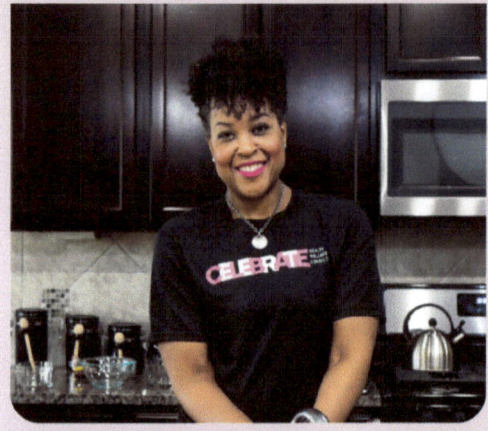

INTEGRATIVE HEALTH & FUNCTIONAL MEDICINE

Are you interested in addressing the root cause of your gut issues? Struggle with low energy, bloating, gas, diarrhea and/or constipation, losing weight, or brain fog?

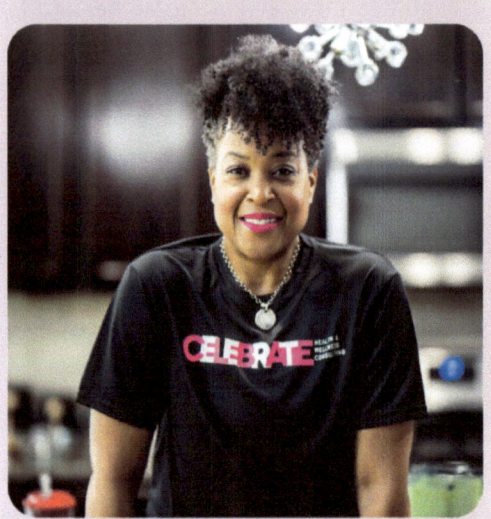

My goal is to help rebalance your body and mind by with Integrative Health & Functional Medicine strategies to feel renewed and rejuvenated again.

For more information, contact Dr. Katashia at info@drkatashia.com to schedule your free consultation.

@drkatashia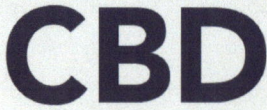

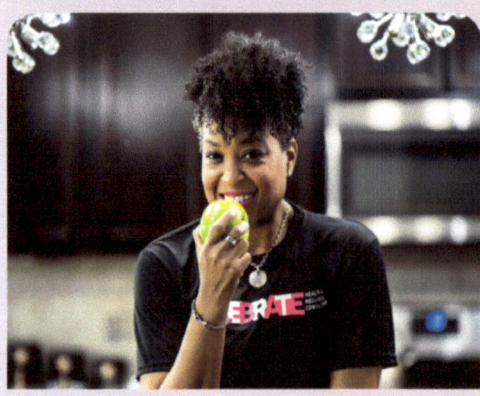

Get Your Pharmacist Approved
CBD

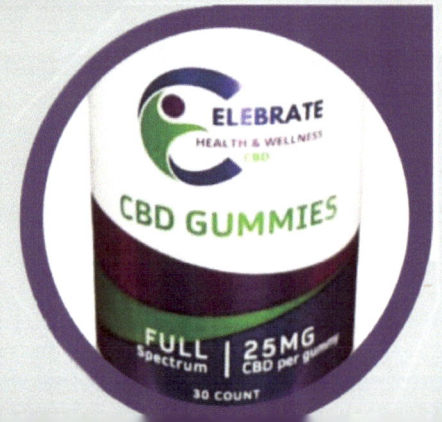
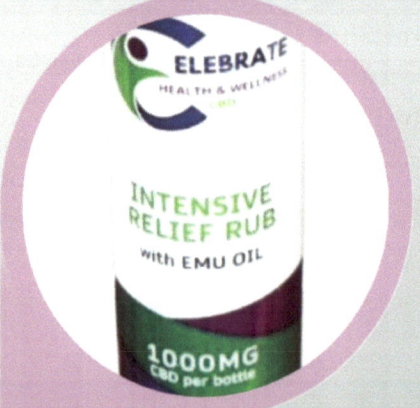
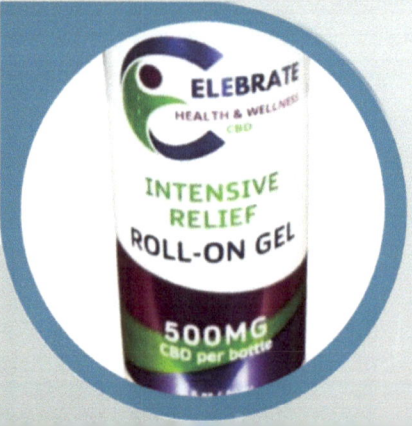

LESSONS IN FERTILITY

BIRTHING POSSIBILITIES

by Dr. Katashia Partee Kendrick

There are many faces of infertility. I am only one of them. Maya Angelou once said, "I may be changed by what happens to me, but I refuse to be reduced by it." At one point in my life, I was ashamed to wear that face but today my older, wiser self has convinced the scared me to be bold because my story just might inspire someone to embrace their journey.

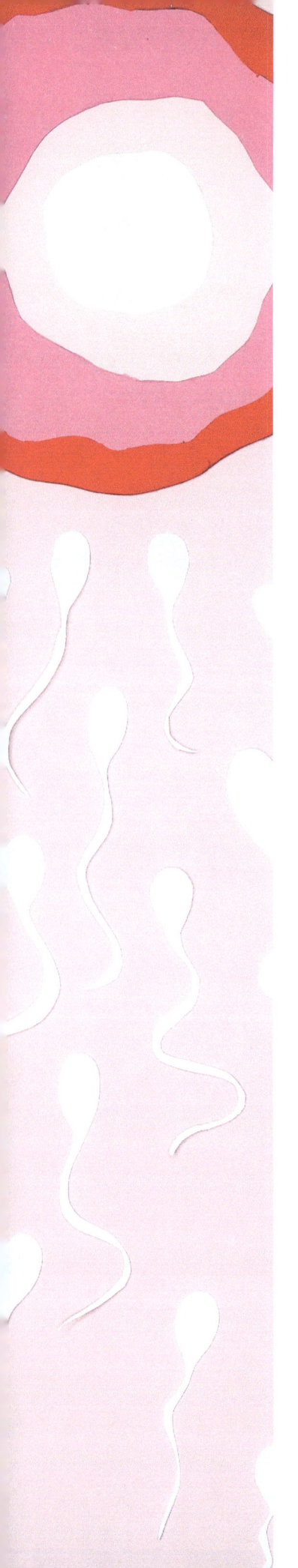

Although I had found the love I once only imagined existed, why was I now paralyzed by pain. Why did my grief overwhelm me at times? I remember in my darkest moments crying inconsolably. Why did my husband and I have to face this kind of hurt? Why did our forever have to include infertility. I cried, I cried and I cried. I asked why had fibroids ravaged my body since my early 20s, inflicting my first myomectomy upon my uterus at the age of 26 then another at the age of 36. Only to endure it all again merely two years later. Why had the fibroids come back and this time with vengeance, literally taking the energy out of me? My daily routine now included blood transfusions and iron infusions due to severe anemia. Then at the age of 38, the darkness surrounded me and I had a hysterectomy. Why would I never know the joy of being pregnant? Why would I never hold in my arms the baby my husband and I had always dreamt of having?

Can I be honest? Transparent even…I was confused! Sad! Broken! I was soooo MAD at GOD. Why did this happen to me? Have you ever had a time in your life when you were mad at GOD? I know I have. But then, look at what God did. In that very moment, GOD had to me remind me that birth can come from other aspects. Along the way, I have received God's message. Have you ever gone through some pain in your life and GOD taught you there is purpose in the pain if you would only receive it? Today, I want to share my lessons learned. You may already have personal knowledge of these lessons but if you would allow me, I would like to share my infertility journey with you today.

LESSON NUMBER ONE

My Creator taught me to have FAITH! It's that simple…FAITH. I was broken… have you ever been broken? I MEAN TRULY BROKEN! My husband and I were hurt. We cried together, we were hurt together, it was always we through all these emotions. We rode the emotional rollercoaster, together.

GOD taught me to have FAITH. Faith that HE can do anything but fail. He didn't fail me. It was not in His plan for me. God is the source of my strength and I needed that strength. I didn't go to work on some days, I didn't eat on some days and I am pretty sure I did not shower on some days. My infertility journey broke me. Being Mad at GOD, I didn't have a desire to go to church anymore. However, one particular Sunday the Holy Spirit spoke to me. Go to Church. I heard it clearly so, I did! Guess what? God is an ontime GOD and He had an ontime message just for me. Rev Tamla Wilson spoke that Sunday and she gave her powerful testimony on her infertility journey and shared how she had been victorious in the battle that sought to destroy her. It was my battle. My war. That message was just for me. She discussed how she was starting a support group/ministry called The Waiting Room. The Waiting Room saved my life! God spoke to me through her. God always provides that ram in the bush. You just have to KEEP THE FAITH! Maybe some of you all are looking to keep the faith in your situation. God's word says in Isaiah 43: 19 (NIV) "See, I am doing a new thing! Now it springs up; do you not perceive it? I am making a way in the wilderness and streams in the wasteland. God is working that thing out for you right now. Don't lose faith. Not now, you are so close. Your breakthrough is coming.

God has no limits but I had to accept the facts! I had to receive in my spirit God's word that says in 2 Corinthians 9: 8 (NIV) "And God is able to bless you abundantly, so that in all things at all times, having all that you need, you will abound in every good work." God wanted me to know that He can birth more than I could ever imagine. This singular focus I once had precluded me from being able to see the endless opportunities God's plan offered for me. To imagine that this life I would birth didn't need to come through me but could still very much be a part of me. I realized I can birth possibilities. I CAN BIRTH…A BUSINESS, A BOOK, BETTER HEATLH & WELLNESS…I can birth whatever GOD assigns to me to BIRTH. It may not have been that child to birth, honestly God has something greater in mind. This birth he imagined for me would make a HUGE impact on the world. The word says in Proverbs 3:5 (NLT) "Trust in the Lord with all your heart; do not depend on your own understanding. Seek His will in all you do, and He will show you which path to take."

LESSON NUMBER THREE…TELL THE TRUTH…TELL YOUR STORY!

I was ashamed of my story. People always asked…when are you going to have a baby? When are you going to start having children? How many of you can relate? Do you know how embarrassing this was for me? Anyone ever been embarrassed by well-meaning family and friends? To know that I wasn't able to give my husband what he desired. I was devastated! However, today I am speaking from my scars and not my wounds. What my husband desired was to be happy and whole with me. Although he would have loved to have been a father, he loved me more. He chose not to focus on what was lacking, he always saw the love. He loved me even when I questioned why he would. I was so focused on what I did not have, I almost missed seeing what God had blessed us with; each other.

Like in Jeremiah 29:11 (NLT) For I know the plans I have for you, "says the Lord". They are plans of good and not for disaster, to give you a future and a hope. GOD taught me by telling my story I just might remind someone else that God has a plan for your life and it is not filled with disaster. Let my story change someone's else life by reminding them of their future filled with hope. Are you listening to this saying…I have a story? Well, whatever your story is…GOD wants you to share it because your story can make a big impact in somebody's life. The word says in Romans 10:17 (NLT), Faith comes from hearing the Good news about Christ. Tell your story.

I wasn't on this journey alone…I had the Lord, of course, my husband and my mom. My husband and my mom always sought to encourage me to look at what God could do and not simply focus on what would never be. They often encouraged me to consider other paths to becoming a mom and although back then I was totally against it, I have since learned how to consider the possibilities. I can birth possibilities. I encourage you as I encourage myself not to give up…to look at alternative options such as adoption. Where once I would have emphatically placed a period, I now place a coma because there is more to be written. My heart has softened and I am open to all that God has in store for the Kendricks.

Just remember, the ugliest and messiest part of your journey will be one of the most powerful parts of your testimony…how you overcame it! Rev Tamla's story and how she overcame changed me forever The Waiting Room continues to give me Hope. My hope now is that my story of how I overcame can encourage you in your walk. I am happy. The broken pieces are now replaced with a sense of peace.

It's a chapter in my life but not your whole story. I am smiling because I know GOD is good and that I am standing on the side of this journey waiting for you. The word says in 1 Corinthians 15:57 (NKJV) "But thanks be to God, who gives us the victory through our Lord Jesus Christ. Won't you join me on the other side.

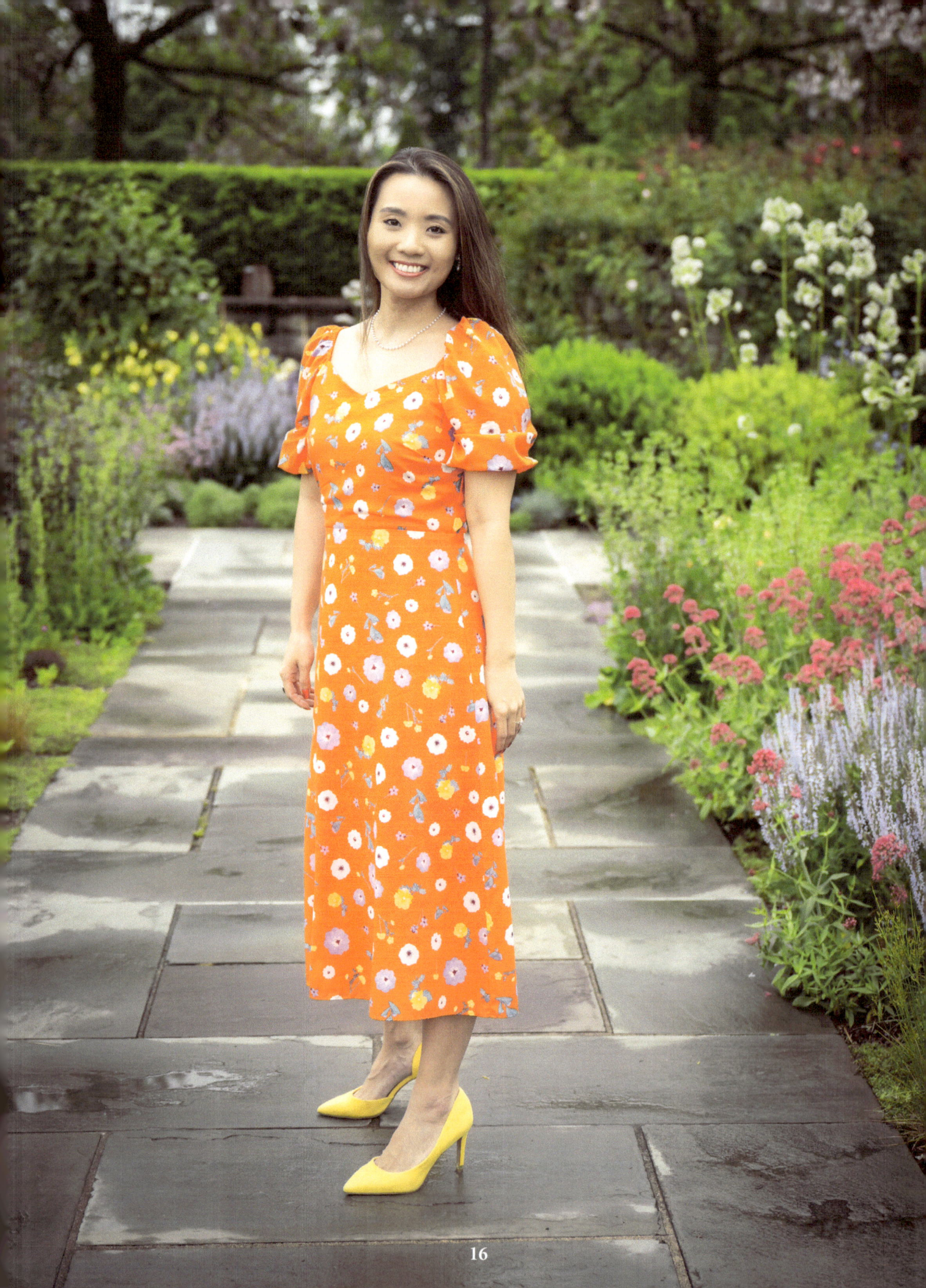

PATIENT SAFETY ANALYST

DR. MYUNGSUN (SUNNY) RO

Be Curious, Dream Big

Tell your story...how did you get here?

As a young immigrant growing up in the USA, I had been repeatedly told that honest, hard work was the only and surest way to succeed in the USA.

And throughout my childhood, the "work hard" mentality worked. The first summer in the USA was spent voluntarily memorizing the entire list of irregular English verb forms from the back of a dictionary. Just 8 years after arriving to the new country, I graduated valedictorian from high school and earned scholarships to attend the college of my dreams, the Johns Hopkins University (JHU) in Baltimore, Maryland, with the goal of becoming a physician.

However, my heart had different plans for me. During my undergraduate years, I was deeply touched by the inequity and the value of community engagement in the beloved city of Baltimore, which inspired me to become a local high school teacher and a behavioral specialist for children with special needs. There, through some of my most heart-wrenching losses and most exhilarating wins, I learned some of the most important lessons of life – of resilience, patience, gratitude, and unconditional love.

When I decided to change my career to healthcare, the pathway didn't turn out so straightforward, either. Despite the university honors and high test scores, years of preparation, and positive assurance from the career advisors, I failed to get accepted into a medical school. That's when I decided to explore the profession of pharmacy and the impact of the pharmacists in healthcare for my Master's thesis, which proved to be one of the best and most pivotal decisions of my life. I learned that pharmacists are among the true educators of healthcare, and the degree could open the door to incredibly diverse pathways, including the

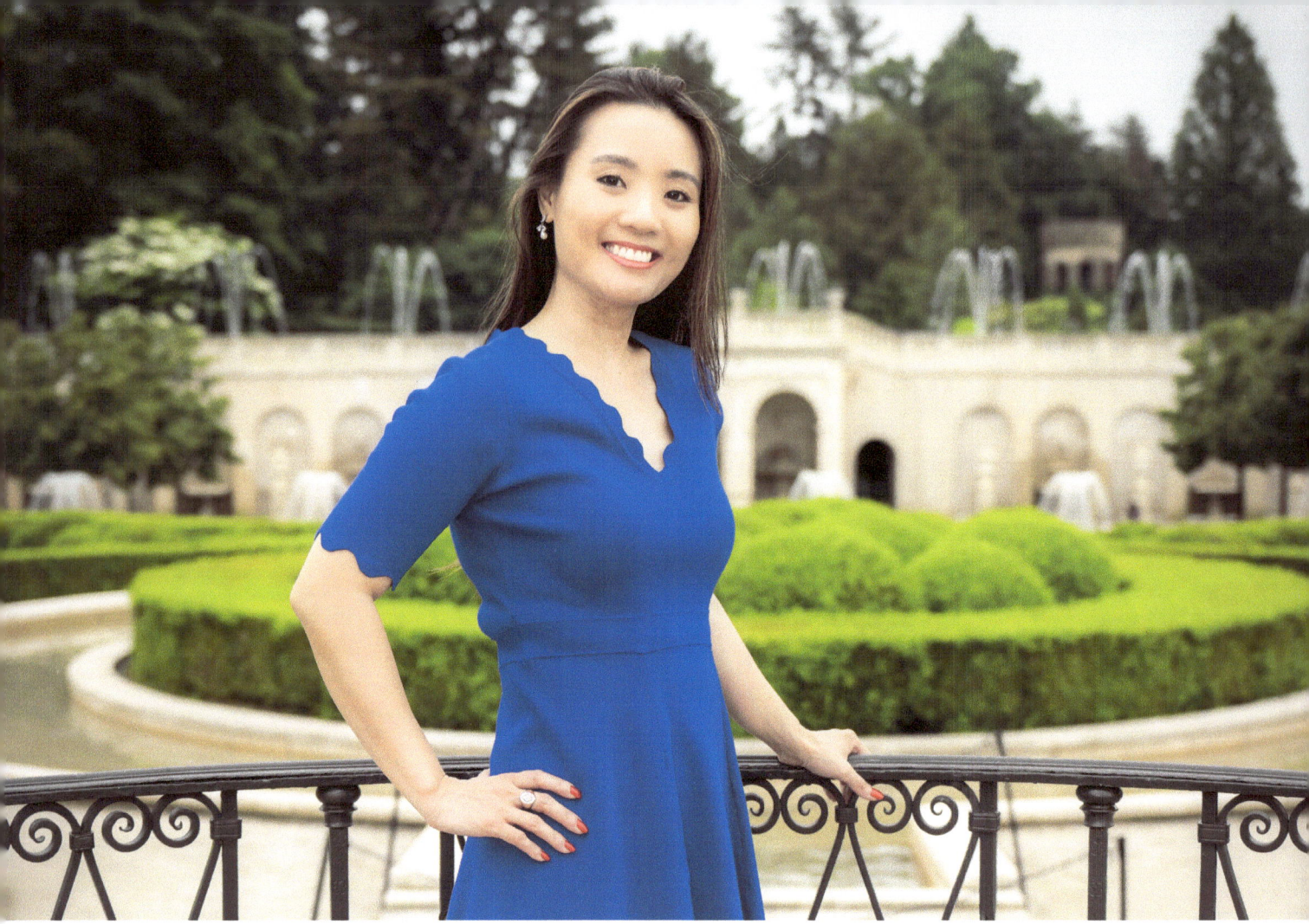

ability to impact patient care both individually and globally.

And just when I thought I finally found the ideal pathway in pharmacy to do just that – by completing a PGY2 residency in medication use safety and policy, again my heart stepped in. Despite my dreams to pursue this particular residency track since my very first year of pharmacy school, I made a difficult last-minute, devastating decision not to apply. I reflected, re-evaluated, and prayed…

Today I am a Patient Safety Analyst at the Pennsylvania Safety Authority (PSA), having completed specialized fellowship training in both medication and patient safety. At PSA I will have the opportunity to analyze error reports from healthcare facilities and institutions across the state of Pennsylvania and write for publication in their journal, Patient Safety. Through my work, I hope to raise awareness on important patient safety topics and touch the lives of many around the world, at both the individual level and the systems level.

The truth is, if you don't follow your heart and get your heart broken several times along the way, you will not learn the most beautiful and vital lessons in life. Resilience, kindness, gratitude, and forgiveness are just as important as "hard work" to achieving success. Let yourself shine, triumphantly, with wins and losses and all, and make the world a step closer to what you WANT it to be, what it SHOULD be.

Are there things that I wish I would've done differently along the way? Probably. But it doesn't

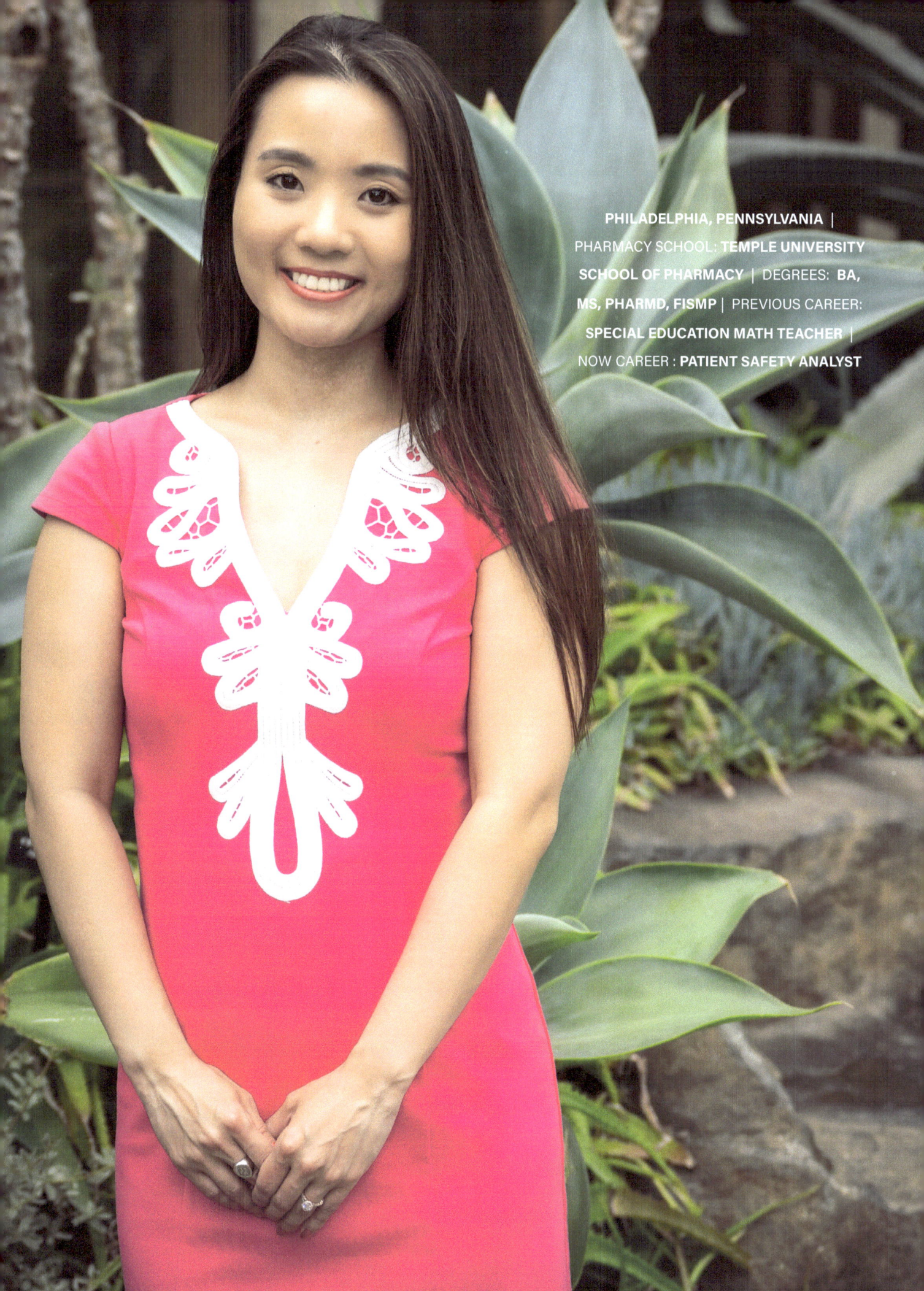

PHILADELPHIA, PENNSYLVANIA | PHARMACY SCHOOL: **TEMPLE UNIVERSITY SCHOOL OF PHARMACY** | DEGREES: **BA, MS, PHARMD, FISMP** | PREVIOUS CAREER: **SPECIAL EDUCATION MATH TEACHER** | NOW CAREER : **PATIENT SAFETY ANALYST**

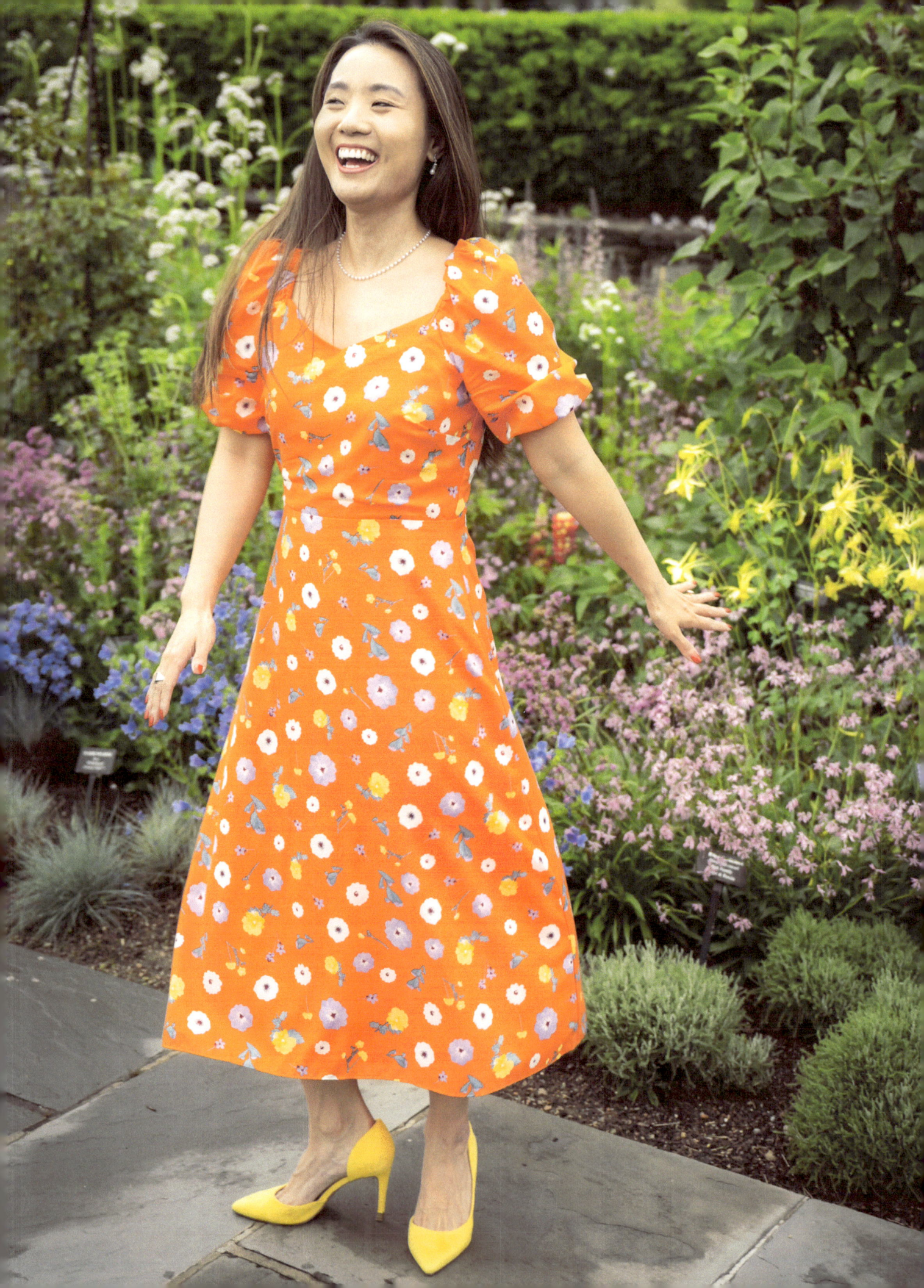

matter. What matters now is the person I am TODAY, and what endless beautiful possibilities TODAY has to unfold.

Describe what you are building/have built (your business; your career)

I am passionate about education and advocacy. My ultimate goal is to spread awareness, inspire change, and unite various members inside and outside the healthcare industry to make patient care safer.

What's been your biggest lesson you have learned along your journey?

I have learned to stand by my truth and set boundaries. When a plan goes awry, all you have to do is forgive yourself and others, learn your lessons and move along, and trust that the universe will take care of the rest.

How do you respond to fear?

When I am facing an unknown, I follow the 10/10/10 rule – and ask myself, how will I feel about this decision in 10 minutes, 10 months, and 10 years? Will I feel immediate satisfaction from this action but regret it down the road? Ten years from now, will I be proud of this decision and all its potential implications?

What does it mean to be considered a leader in your profession and industry?

My philosophy is to lead with heart, with both passion and COMpassion. More specifically, in this chapter of my life, my goal is to lead with an honest, empathetic, and unrelenting voice that can touch many hearts and inspire change in healthcare through education and advocacy.

At this time, pharmacists are being challenged to think out of the box more than ever. What advice do you have for the pharmacist who is wondering how to do that?

Let failure be your biggest lesson and others' doubt your biggest motivation! Don't settle with others' expectations of you – be curious and dream big.

Who do you look up to or model yourself after (personal or professional)?

The biggest role models in my life are those who are the closest to me, including my husband, family, and friends. I firmly believe in the adage that "we are who we walk with" and I am grateful to be surrounded by those who consistently challenge me, shower me with love, show me lifelong lessons, and be my rock of support.

What message would you share with other colleagues in pharmacy?

Never take any opportunity for granted. Constantly seek new knowledge, cultivate relationships, and use your failures as a springboard to create something better every day, including a better YOU.

What's next for you and/or your business?

Upon the completion of my fellowship programs I will be starting a new position as the Patient Safety Analyst at the Pennsylvania Patient Safety Authority, with a focus on medication safety. I hope to add valuable new information and contribute to important discussions surrounding patient safety based on analysis of literature and error reports.

Where can we find you to further connect? (no email addresses or phone numbers please)

LinkedIn, X

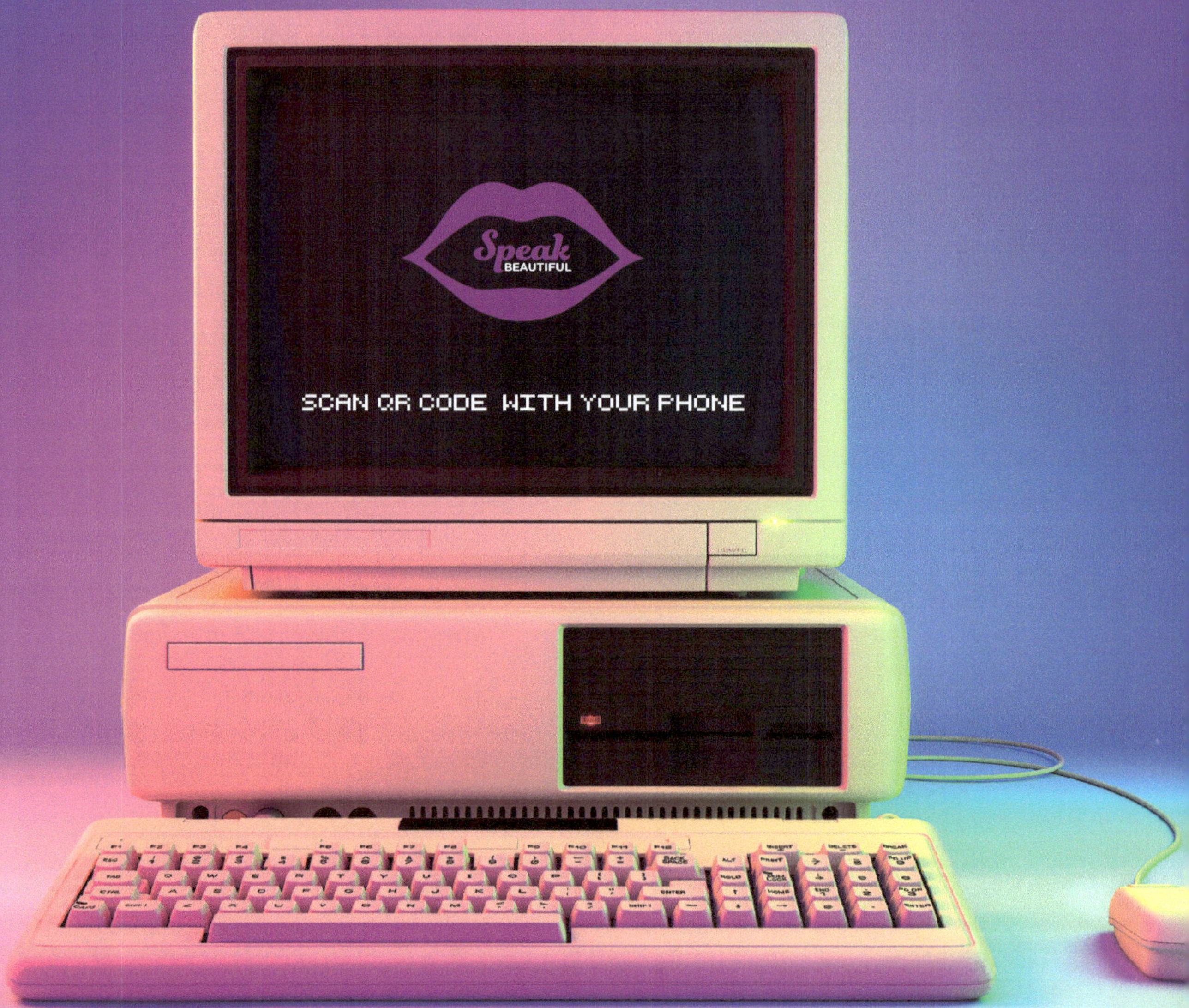

THINK BEYOND.

Speak Beautiful is where passion and innovation meet to bring your ideas to life for marketing, brand, and product design. We are dedicated to converting your vision into reality with fresh perspectives on how to extend your reach. Our agency understands the needs of every size client and provides top-of-the-line service with passion and over 20+ years experience. We are your one-stop shop for your end-to-end design needs.

SCAN TO EXPERIENCE

SPEAKBEAUTIFUL.COM

GRAPHIC DESIGN | PACKAGING | TRADESHOW AND EVENT DESIGN | WEBSITE DEVELOPMENT | TV AND FILM

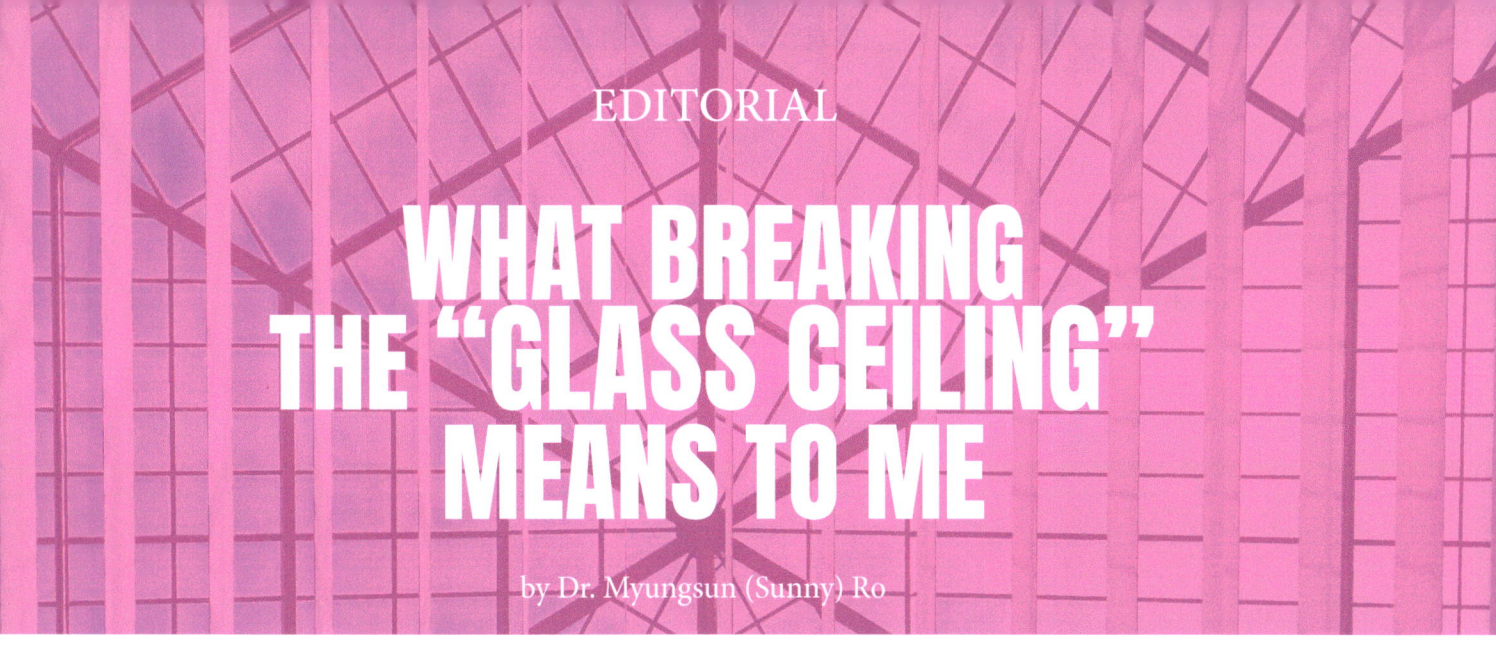

EDITORIAL

WHAT BREAKING THE "GLASS CEILING" MEANS TO ME

by Dr. Myungsun (Sunny) Ro

For as long as I can remember, as I wholeheartedly strived to personify the "work hard and you'll succeed" mentality, my understanding of the term "glass ceiling" had been rather simplistic and elusive: implicit barriers that women and members of minorities face in professional advancement. In other words, if you're the first in your community or demographic population to achieve a particular goal, then you have successfully broken the glass ceiling.

However, in my experience as an immigrant, the first in my family to earn a doctorate degree in the USA, and a pharmacist in a non-traditional career, my encounter with the "glass ceiling" turned out to be much more complex, pervasive, and surprisingly, ingrained.

First, when you're the first person to pave a new trail, you may not have the support of mentors and supporters who can fully relate to your unique background, aspirations, and challenges. At some point in your career, you may suddenly realize that the guidance from your trusted mentor may no longer be relevant to your singularly unique experience, leaving you to forge new ideas, seek additional sources of knowledge, and simply learn from your own failures.

Next and perhaps the most well-known aspect of the glass ceiling is the implicit and explicit bias from others "outside" the glass. What was unbeknownst to me, however, was the phenomenon that when an unfounded assumption is made by another, it is sometimes because the perpetrator is seeing his or her own reflection in the glass, not you. Therefore, what others perceive of you may actually be unintended projections of their own unresolved issues. When people encounter a unicorn for the first time, or something that they do not fully understand, some may take the easy route of drawing preconceived conclusions from their narrow personal schemas rather than taking the steps to get to know the real you. And remember, hurt people hurt people.

One of the most challenging aspects of the glass ceiling, to me, was breaking my own family's generational cycle and taking a leap of faith that your family may not approve of or even understand. Despite their best intentions, they may carry a limited, outdated, or foreign mentality that prioritizes security, stability, and conformity. Even worse, some of these ideas may be indoctrinated from an early age, which may be almost impossible to break.

Lastly, sometimes we are our own worst enemy. Impostor syndrome claims too many women in the workplace, debilitating our own ability to see ourselves clearly and rise confidently. We need to understand that it is okay to make mistakes, that our failures can serve as valuable lessons, and that we need to move on swiftly, because we may be the *only* ones down the road who are still dwelling on it.

The idea of "glass ceiling" turned out to be a construct built by not just those outside the glass, but also from within. And it has the unfortunate tendency to mirror those who look into it, projecting the worst reflections of our own selves onto what we see. Therefore, for all of the pioneers and innovators trying to shatter the glass ceiling – next time, look within. There lies the most elusive and toughest of all – yourself.

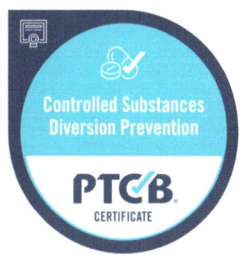 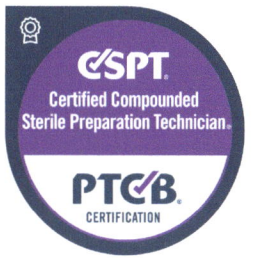

FOCUS ON STYLE

The Heart and Mind of *Style*

A Stylish Conversation with Dr. Danielle and Elle Renée

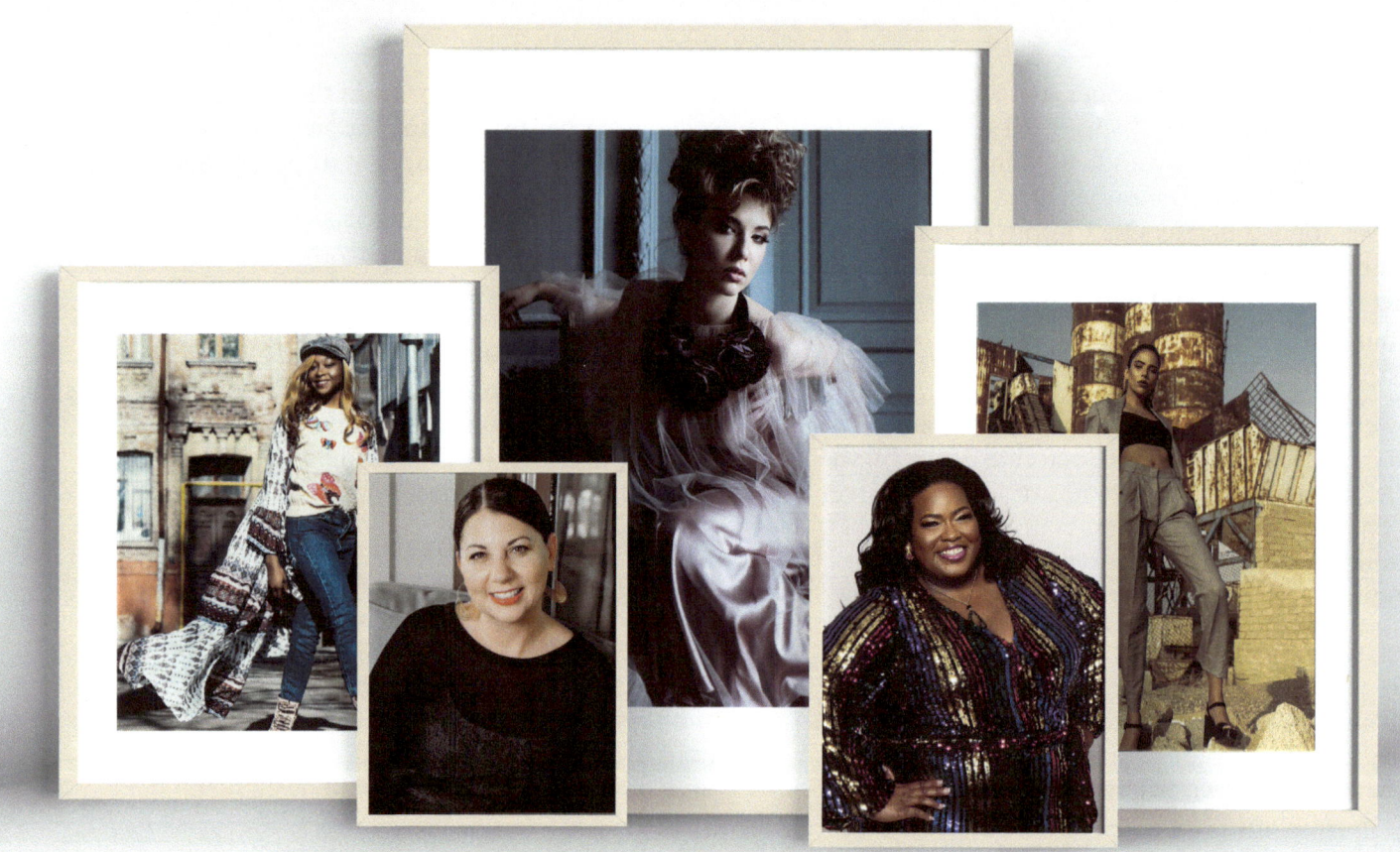

Do you know two women who are both pharmacists, who have a passion for fashion and love helping others discover their style? If not, you do now. Meet Dr. Danielle Perrodin and Dr. Leslie Hodge (also known as Elle Renée), two Doctors of Pharmacy who offer different recommendations to cure the styling woes that women often face.

Just like medicine, there is no one style fits all, but these two women in pharmacy and fashion have figured out the prescription of success that works best for them and their clients. In a candid conversation about the heart and mind of style, Dr. Danielle and Elle Renée discussed their experiences that lead to them the fashion forward women they are today.

Elle Renée: *How important is mindset when it comes to image and branding oneself?*

Danielle: I believe mindset is everything, so of course it is going to be important when you are creating your brand and your image. I really believe it is an important thing to consider before you create anything because the mindset that you create from is going to dictate the result of what you create. So that is why I really work with my clients to unveil the limiting beliefs that are within their mindset and create those beliefs that are going to support the brand and the image that they want. As a result, I also feel that the brand and image can only be from a place of total authenticity. So, I do not believe that you can create a successful brand or image out of being fake or trying to be like someone else, or having feelings of unworthiness, and trying to create from that space.

Elle Renée: *Where did your passion for fashion come from and who were some of your inspirations when it came to finding your own style?*

Danielle: I can remember as a little girl playing with barbie dolls and paper dolls and the sketch outfits, but I think it was in my DNA from my dad's side. My grandmother had the most beautiful costume jewelry, and so did my aunt. She always had the best clothes and this amazing style. She mostly shopped thrift stores and consignments. As a teenager, I preferred new clothes but now I'm learning to appreciate more of how she created her style through that aspect. My mom also influenced me. Her style was very neat and practical. She ironed everything! I hate to iron, but I do I think my style comes from her as well. I was also inspired by Audrey Hepburn and Marilyn Monroe, that old World Classic, yet a little bit of sexy, fun and playful.

Elle Renée: *What is your favorite type of client or characteristics of an ideal client?*

Danielle: My favorite client is women in pharmacy, and I even go narrower than that to women in pharmacy that are trying to create something that make a big impact on the world, that have a holistic approach to changing the health care system. Most of them are creating an online functional medicine business and want to attract clients. I help them to dress as their highest self, build a brand and improve their image so that they can grow their business. The reason I love working with holistic wellness leaders is because of the mind set work I share with them. Most have had experience with or have been exposed to some of the tools and resources that I do share with them and they're more open to it.

Elle Renee: *What should every woman invest in when in, when it comes to pieces of clothing?*

Danielle: Every woman should absolutely invest in great undergarments. And I'll tell you why. It really is the foundation. What you wear under your clothes, really determines on how you feel, and if you're wearing undergarments that make you feel not really so great, it's going to show. A lot of women believe that no one sees it, so then they keep wearing the same...worn out, ugly, ill-fitting undergarments...forever. They are just afraid to invest in more pieces or they think it doesn't matter because no one sees it... but guess what, they do see it. They see it in your confidence and how you feel. A great fitting pair of panties and a bra that has been properly sized for your body today, not your body 10 years ago, can really make or break your fashion sense.

Elle Renée: *What specialized training or certifications have you pursued to elevate your services and offerings?*

Danielle: I became certified with Kate Taylor Certified Style School and her Virtual Style Mastery, and still learning through Business of Style. Learning how to virtually style people because when I started this business in 2019, it was right before the pandemic, and no one could have imagined that everyone would be moving to all online. And it just really opened up for me to be able to work with women across the globe. I had one style client that was in Costa Rica when I worked with her. Another client was visiting in Kenya for one of our calls. I have clients that are across the country. and in fact, most of my clients are not located in Louisiana. I am part of the Hue and Stripe community which gives me access to some of the best stylists in the world as a resource. Just recently, And you and I, Leslie, had taken a certification together with Love E Fashion back in 2019, I believe. That was super fun to do that with you. We learned so much about the whole area of fashion. I continue to sponsor Acadiana Fashion Week every year, I gain so much knowledge just being in that venue. I am always looking for other certifications and continuing education. Just like in pharmacy.

Elle Renée: *Why is having a business coach important?*

Dr. Danielle: It's so important to hire a business coach because they can see your blind spots. We all have our own blind spots and guess what, we can't see them. And so, when you hire someone to help you, they can save you so much time and effort. Just by holding up a mirror to you and showing you these blind spots. It was so funny when I worked with Dr. Jerrica Dodd, she showed me mine. I remember she once told me, "You need to stop wearing flowers!" At first, I was a little offended. I was like, but I love my flowers. It's my style. But, you know, once I committed to slowly weaned myself off of the floral prints, it opened me up to all of the other designs that I was saying no to. I think this lesson could apply to anyone with any type of business coach. You have what you're used to and familiar with and the coach might take that away from you. Show you a different way, and sometimes that different way is so much better than you can even imagine. But as the coaches their job is to have that vision for you. They are the visionary. They can see a couple miles down the road when you're just in it and all you can see is what's happening to you right here and right now.

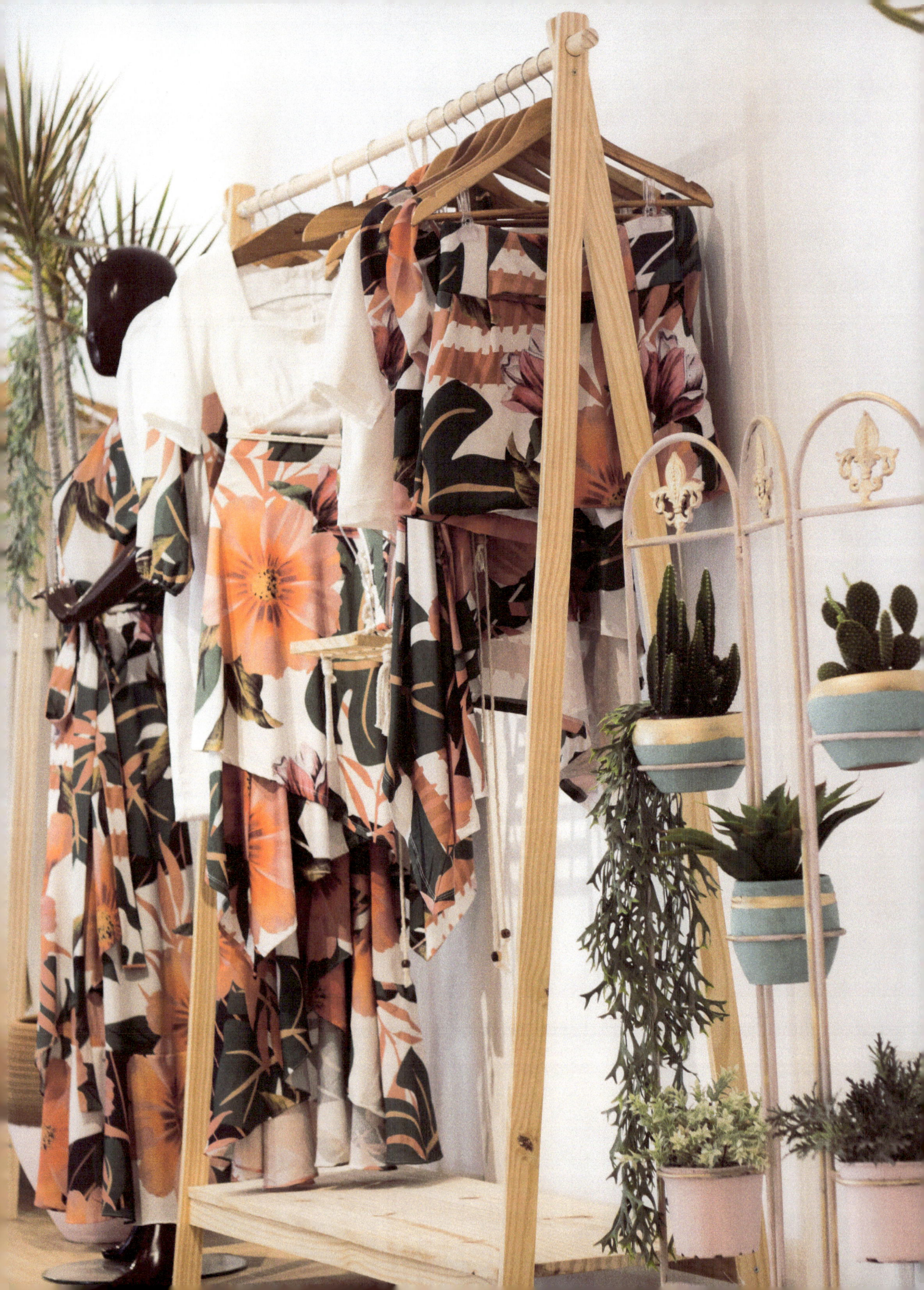

Elle Renee: *What is your favorite accessory to wear and why?*

Danielle: So, I'm not big on accessories, believe it or not. I am very minimalistic, but I do like to accessorize, and I think it's important. But my very favorite accessory to wear are my hexagon shaped gold earrings. I believe it is because it just reminds me of where I come from. It reminds me of my love of science and reminds me of my love of biochemistry. I am showing my nerdy side, but it just it makes me feel like myself. I am not trying to be someone else. It is a nod to who I am, what I love and they just make me feel really good about myself. They are not flashy but they're interesting and I think it says a lot about my own personal style.

Elle Renee: *What is your favorite place to shop and why?*

Danielle: I have just discovered a new favorite place to shop, and the reason is because I am focusing more and more on creating a capsule wardrobe that's more sustainable and eco-friendly. The shop is VETTA and not only are the pieces there sustainable, but some are convertible and reversible. So, if you're only going to only have a select number of items in your wardrobe, wouldn't it behoove you to have items that you can easily wear in different ways? The tops and dresses can be worn front or backwards for different styles. And the fabrics are reversible to change up the color or pattern. So, I think it is really brilliant, and I am enjoying that right now.

Elle Renee: *How has being an image consultant allowed you to help inspire and support other women owned businesses?*

Danielle: I really have enjoyed all these questions Leslie. I love collaborating. I've been doing that since the beginning, but I think the way that I've helped other business owners was really by being a role model. I love Human Design and my profile is 6/2, which is the role model. I do that by showing up online consistently talking about my business, making offers, being my true authentic. I encourage them that they too can create something new and different out of nothing other than their gifts and talents. I support them by emphasizing how important it is to get great branding photos. One of the easiest ways to grow your business is to share high-quality photos that show your face. And what better way to do that than to invest in a stylist for your photoshoot!

Danielle: *How did you first know you wanted to be a stylist?*
Elle Renée: I love fashion and helping people create looks from items they already have in their closet or if we were shopping together, seeing how they really transform when they put something on that they like or really complemented their figure or complexion or just their overall desired look. I just love that, and so I didn't know that I wanted to be a stylist per se I just know I enjoyed fashion, I enjoyed clothes, jewelry, shoes, all types of accessories and how you can literally transform how you feel by spending extra time into creating a look.

Danielle: *OK I love your style business name I think I may have told you this before but I once had a dog named Hoosier daddy so it really resonated with me. What made you choose that name other than it being very catchy?*

Elle Renée: I think you did tell me about your dog which is so funny because we actually have a place down here called a Hoosier doggy. I think the name came while on a coaching group call and I was just talking about styling and what I wanted to call it. I actually started off calling my company at the time when I first launched – WEAR YOU and then while I remember being on the call I can't remember the reason why but it was myself, Jerrica and a few other people were in a coaching group and I said I wanted to create looks where others would say Who's Your Stylist? And when I said it I was like wait…Hoosier, Indiana…and so that's where that comes from since I am from Indiana.

Danielle: *I want to know was I a difficult client when you first styled me for my Spring issue of PharmaSIS magazine?*

Elle Renée: Not difficult at all, great question. I had to laugh, if anything it challenged me because if you remember, but I sent you a lot of colorful pieces. The tops were bright and bold and could almost lose you with your small frame so it's funny that my initial take was I know some colors I was just thinking about how I wanted you to feel when you saw yourself featured in the magazine and all I envisioned was color jumping off the page. And so, I think it was a challenge for me because I had to push past what I had envisioned for you without ever speaking to you and really see what you wanted. I had to really think like what does she want, let's factor in how these pictures will be used where they would be used and so of course you were amazing…but difficult, no, not at all. Our experience was very much needed to help me grow so I count it as one of those great opportunities where we start with one thing and get something totally different at the end.

Danielle: *I want to know, what gave you the confidence to create your own pharmacy technician training academy and what was the reason behind it?*

Elle Renée: The confidence to do it really stemmed from the desire to do something that would allow me to personally impact someone but also leave another mark on the profession and so interestingly enough when I was approached to even consider or I should say had I ever thought about opening my own training school I had never thought about that. I always saw it from a standpoint of me working for someone or me coming alongside someone who's already been trained or licensed or whatever but never in a million years had I imagined my own school. The confidence came when I realized teaching was what I had been doing my whole pharmacy career. We just call it management.

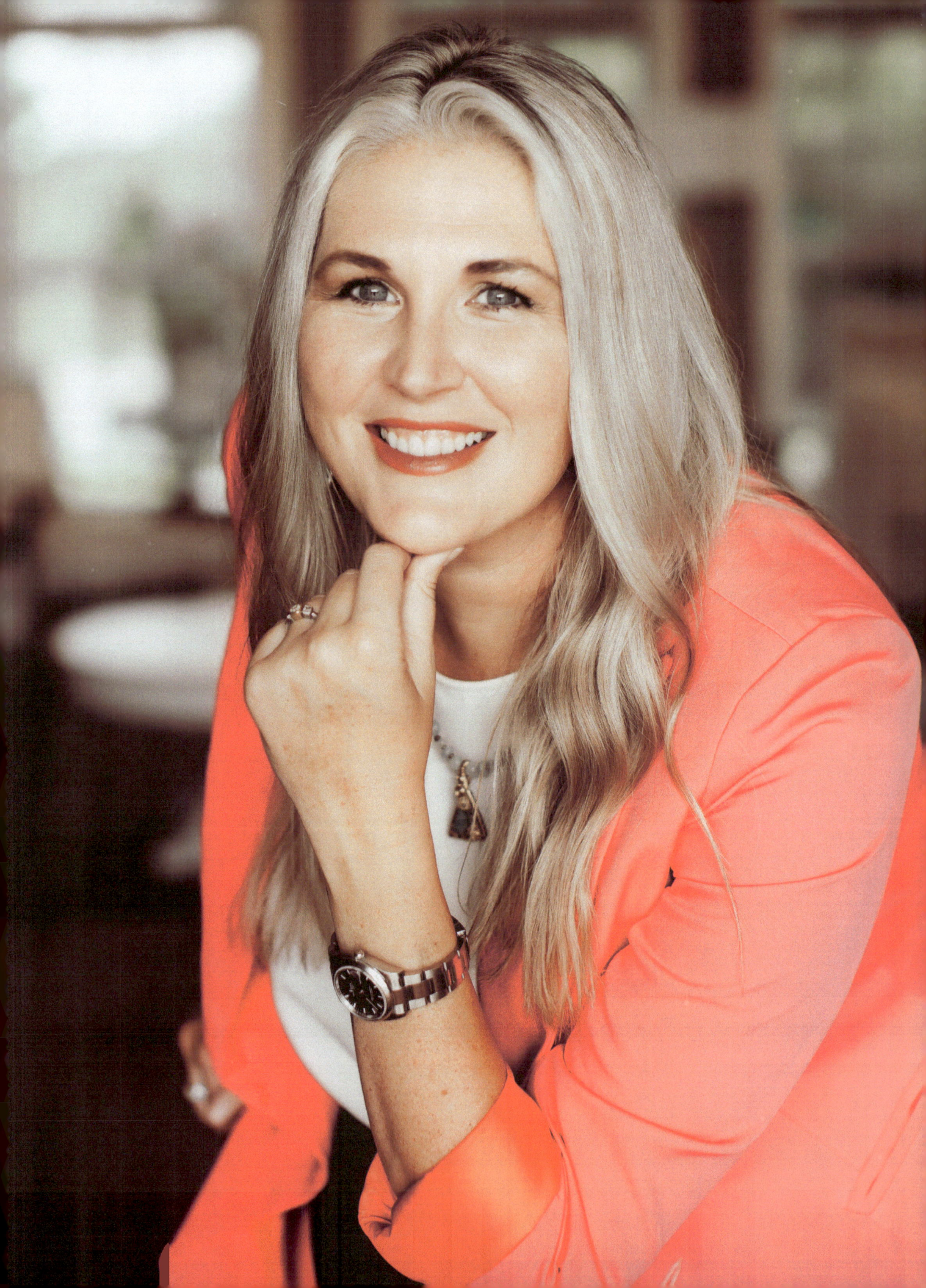

WHERE ARE THEY NOW

DR. BLAIR THIELEMIER
Beyound Your Comfort Zone

POCAHONTAS, ARKANSAS | PHARMACY SCHOOL: **UNIVERSITY OF ARKANSAS FOR MEDICAL SCIENCES** | DEGREES: **PHARMD** | PREVIOUS CAREER: **HOSPITAL AND MTM CONSULTING** | NOW CAREER : **PHARMACY BUSINESS DEVELOPMENT CONSULTANT**

Tell us more of your story...So what happened next?

So much has happened since I first appeared on the cover of the PharmaSis Magazine in 2019. A new baby, a global pandemic, two new businesses! I am still passionate about advancing the profession of pharmacy, however my approach has changed. One of my main focuses today is bringing interprofessional groups of healthcare leaders together in order to have bold and positive conversations about the future of healthcare. There is so much broken in the healthcare system and I believe it is the healthcare professionals standing in their truth that can turn things around. For years we've been saying pharmacy is at a crossroads and thankfully, we are beginning to see forward progress catalyzed by the role pharmacists played in the COVID-19 pandemic. My goals for the future include being a voice for pharmacists in the entrepreneurship and wellness communities as well as seeking new opportunities for pharmacists to leverage their knowledge of biochemistry and cellular metabolism to integrate lifestyle modifications as well as pharmaceutical and natural products use into our standard of practice. I was honored to be named one of the most influential pharmacists in the United States and take my role as a voice for pharmacy very seriously. In my career moving forward, I will continue working with female healthcare consultants through virtual coaching as well as in person retreats at our new retreat center in Costa Rica. Bringing healthcare professionals together for a week of healing and personal growth is my focus for 2023. Entrepreneurship has been one of the biggest blessings of my life and I intend to share.

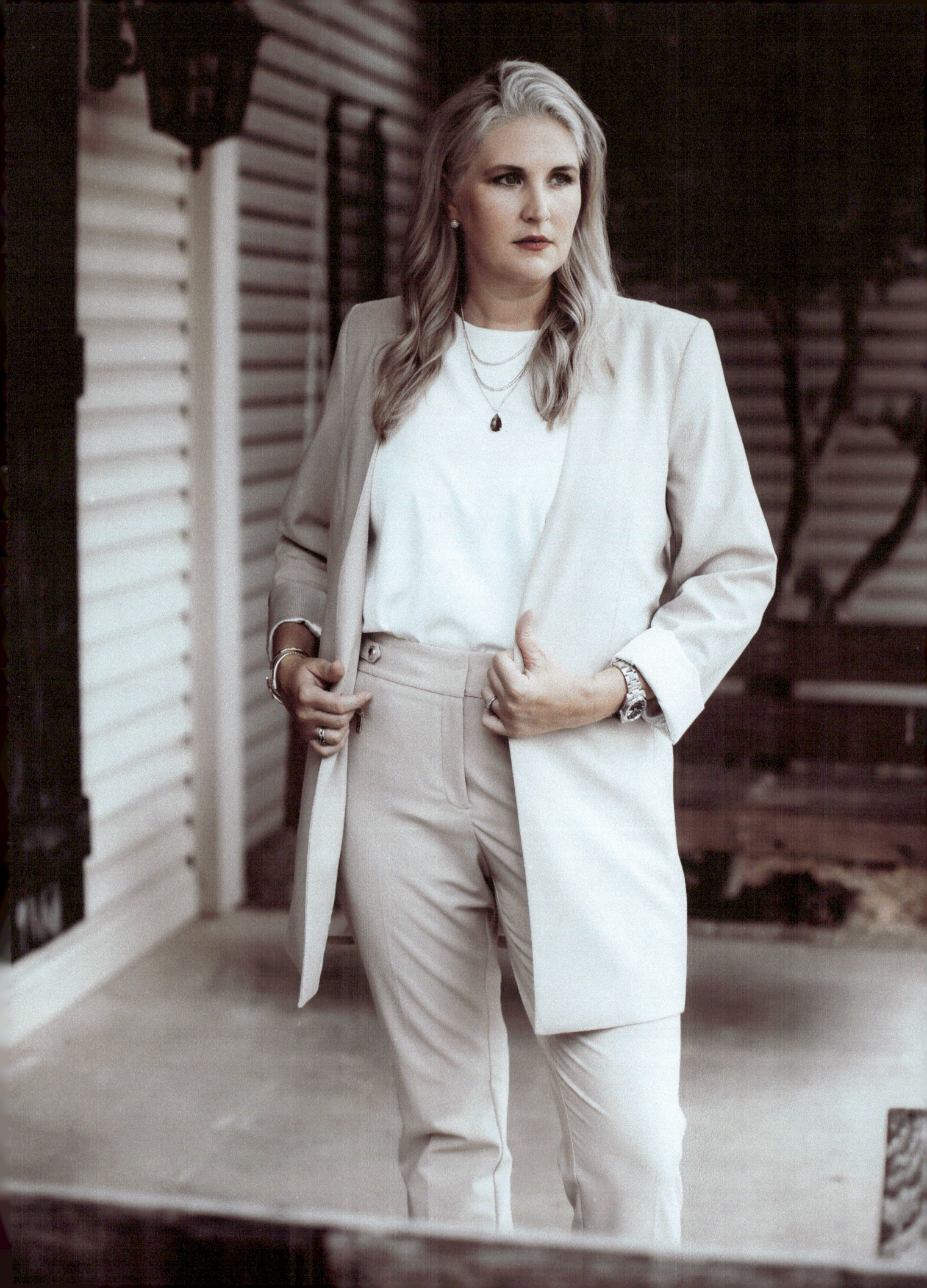

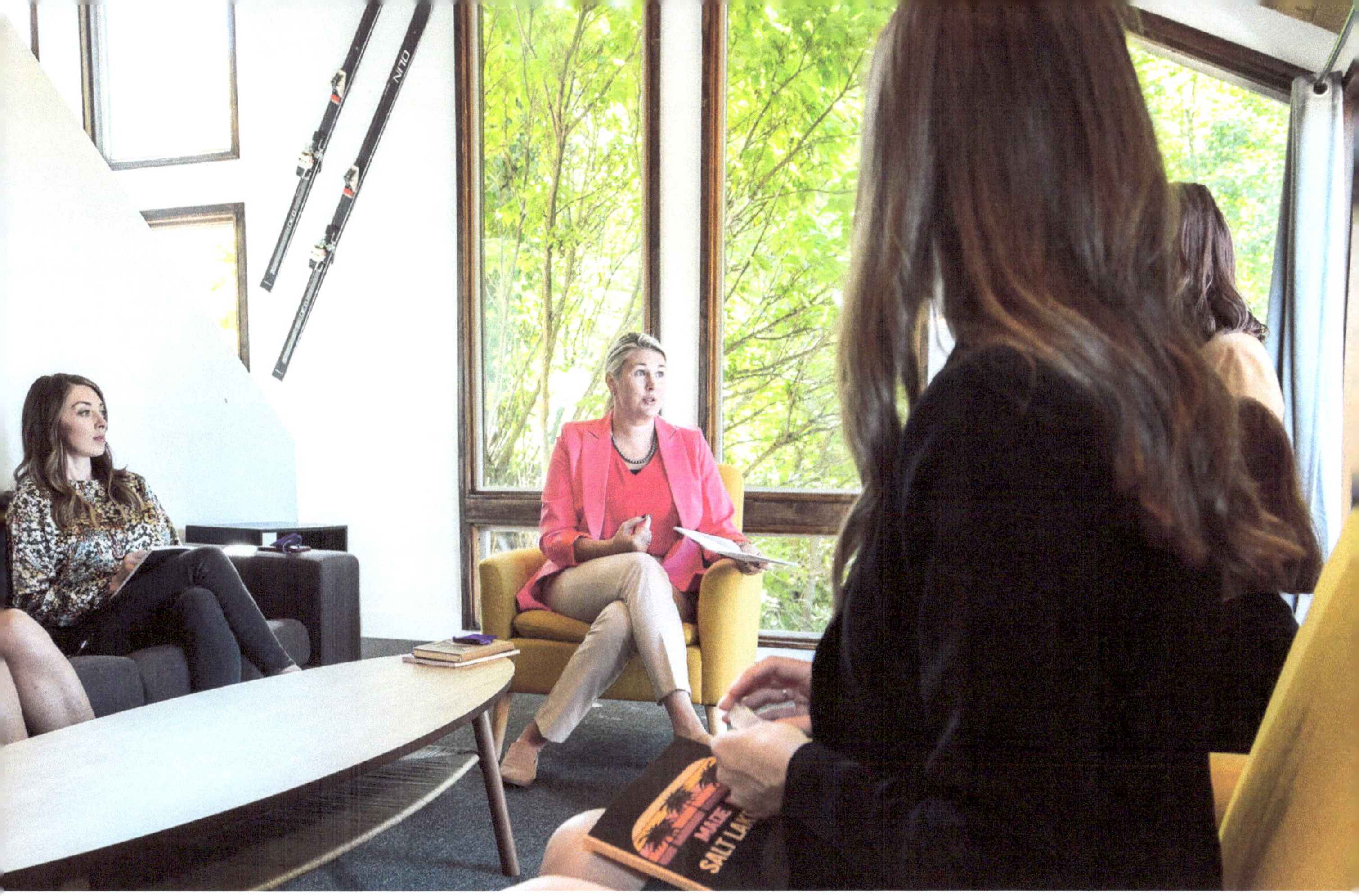

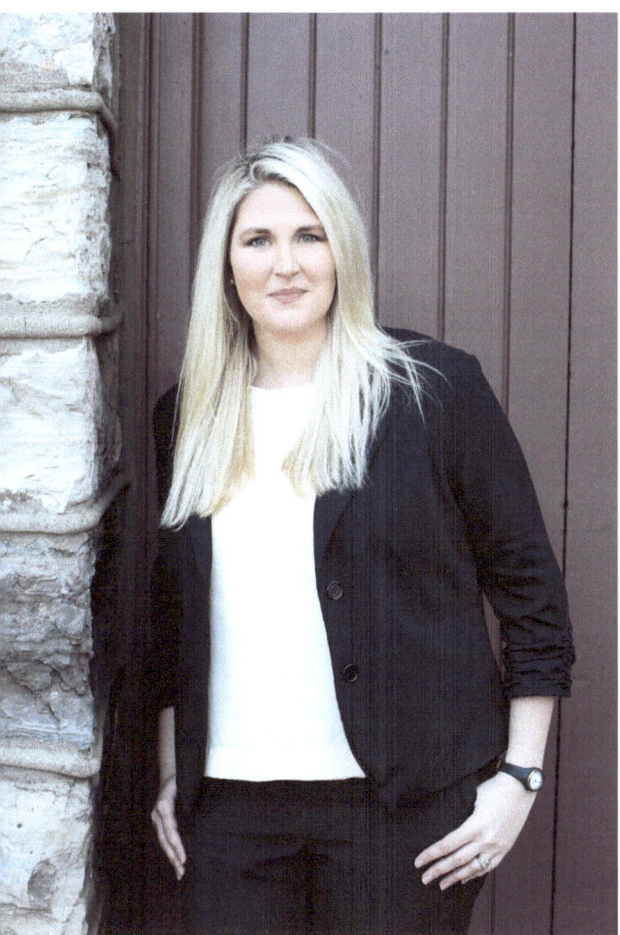

What section of the PharmaSis Magazine were you originally featured?

Spring 2020

How were you featured in the magazine?

Contributing Author

What's new since you last appeared in PharmaSis Magazine?

A lot has changed since I was on the cover in 2020, the world, my family, my marriage, everything transformed. But in a good way! In a way that I intended, because I finally was able to get super clear and super connected to my vision. My vision is to connect holistic and allopathic medicine in a new heart-centered model that promotes healing and compassion.

Any advice for Women in Pharmacy that you would like to share:

The answers to your questions are beyond your comfort zone.

Learning to Battle Self-Criticism

Written By: Dr. Janhavi Punyarthi

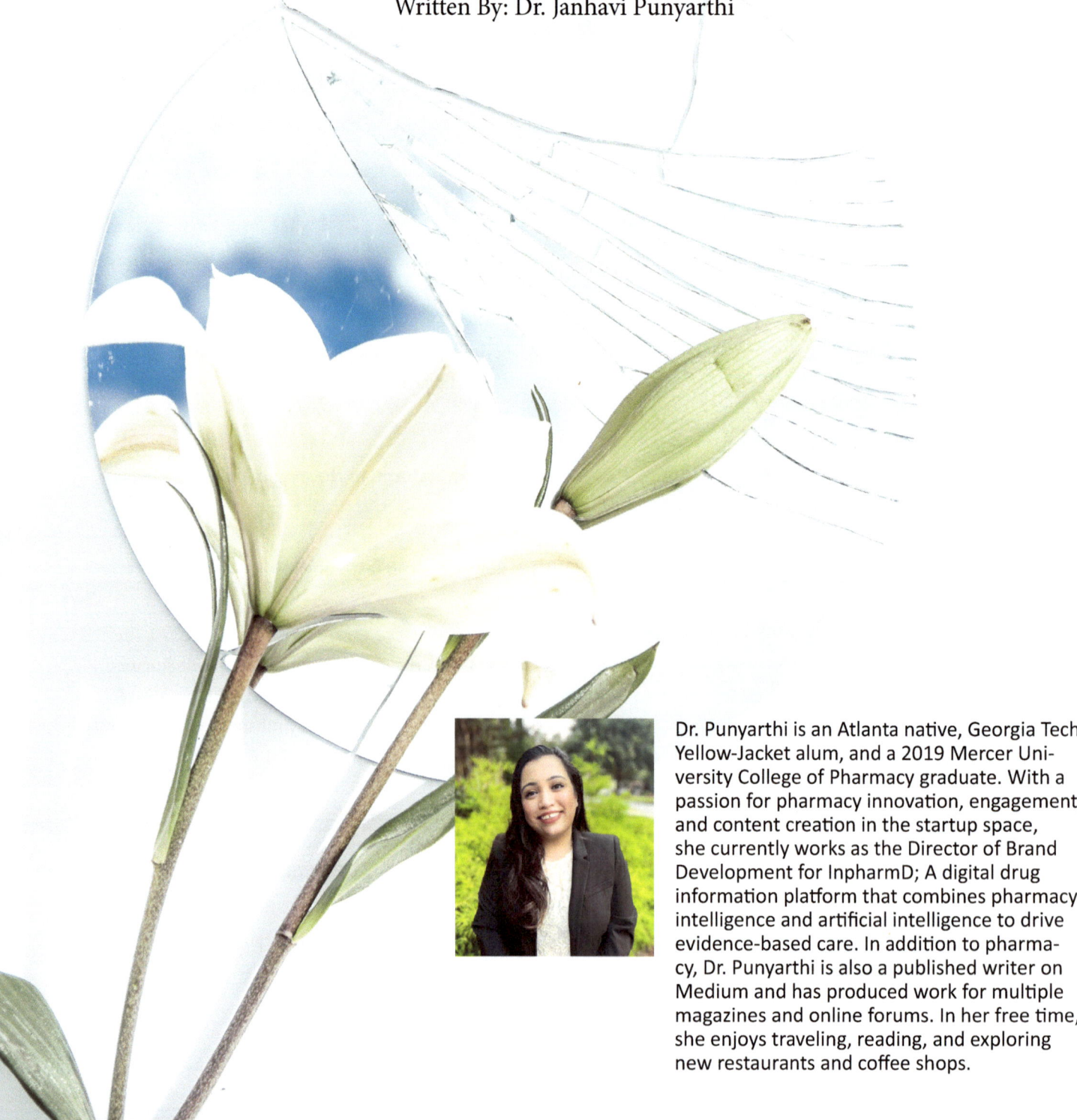

Dr. Punyarthi is an Atlanta native, Georgia Tech Yellow-Jacket alum, and a 2019 Mercer University College of Pharmacy graduate. With a passion for pharmacy innovation, engagement, and content creation in the startup space, she currently works as the Director of Brand Development for InpharmD; A digital drug information platform that combines pharmacy intelligence and artificial intelligence to drive evidence-based care. In addition to pharmacy, Dr. Punyarthi is also a published writer on Medium and has produced work for multiple magazines and online forums. In her free time, she enjoys traveling, reading, and exploring new restaurants and coffee shops.

There's a voice. Sometimes, that voice is vicious. It echoes and booms at me. Other times, it takes on a slier tone, whispering its damage slowly. That sinister voice. It picks at my confidence, tears away at my determination, and makes me question *every single thing*.

"You're not good enough…"

Or worse, "That was good, *but…*"

There's always a stipulation with that voice. There's always a *but*.

It questions and questions and questions. It questions me until I break.

And as my confidence shatters around me, I realize that screeching voice is none other than my own.

Excessive self-criticism is toxic. And for many women in pharmacy, we tend to self-criticize more than most.

As women in pharmacy, we tend to hold ourselves to an extraordinarily high standard. Many of us are high achievers. Many of us chase excellence. And in doing so, we create a set of exorbitantly high, sometimes unattainable expectations.

Perfection must be attained. Satisfactory is not allowed. No middle ground. Excellence or nothing.

The funny thing is that the majority of the time we manage to succeed at our goals. We successfully complete the deliverables and then some. We don't only chase excellence, we catch it.

But even while holding excellence in our bare hands, that voice rears its ugly head, and we crumble.

WHERE DOES SELF-CRITICISM COME FROM?

There is no one answer for this. For some, that self-critical mentality may stem from unresolved trauma. For others, it may be a result of generational behaviors, upbringing, and/or culture.

Often, experiences or patterns in one's past can create insecurity, leading to an increase in self-critical thoughts.

So, insecurity may drive the criticism. But what drives the insecurity?

A huge part of insecurity can stem from the toxic effects of professional social media. Don't get me wrong – there's a lot of good that can come from these outlets as well. However, many times, these platforms normalize unattainable perfection.

These platforms can drive self-criticism. They can create competition and uncertainty. They can create an idealized version of a goal or standard that is realistically unattainable. These glamorized ideals on-screen create a gap between who we feel we are and the idealized version of what we want to be.

The results are damaging: feelings of shame and low self-worth through comparison can become internalized. The critical voice resting at the back of my head begins to shout down the confidence my achievements and determination have earned.

SO HOW DO WE FIX IT?

To be honest, I don't have a perfect answer. I struggle with that voice every day.

But I'm getting better at it. I'm learning to recognize that I'm my own worst critic, and that it's in my hands to tame the voice in my head.

It's not always easy. For years, I've learned to be hyper-aware of my mistakes. I've learned to be self-critical, to question myself, and to always find a flaw. Unlearning toxicity is not immediate nor simple. It's a work in progress, and it requires heaps of concentration and determination.

It begins by recognizing the toxicity. Feedback is not only important; it's essential. Self-work is essential. Criticism, if constructive, is essential.

But when does constructive feedback turn into damaging self-talk? Where do we draw the line?

A good way to start is by removing the stipulations. Instead of saying "*This* was good, but *that* could have been better", change up the language.

That could have been different. *This* was good. *This* being good is not dependent on *that*. *This* was good, full stop!

Secondly, we should increase our awareness of social media toxicity. Maybe, just maybe, if we are more cognizant about the effects of social media on ourselves, we can find a way to limit the damage involved. The first step is realizing that real life is never going to match up to the idealized social-media version in your head. If you choose to ceaselessly compare yourself to a picture-perfect media-world, you choose to be on a treadmill racing to nowhere.

And lastly, we should learn to celebrate the small wins. Battle that toxicity by celebrating ourselves. Many times, we focus on our failures. Many times, we focus on big life goals. We overlook the small wins.

We need to change that. We need to learn to value the little victories.

Self-criticism is a soul-sucking vortex of negativity. Celebrating the smallest of goods in the worst of days shoots a ray of positivity into that vortex and can do wonders for your mental health.

Like I said, it's not easy. There are days when that voice is screaming in my head, until I'm a miserable shell, calling myself a failure over and over again.

But, I'm trying. I'm learning to celebrate myself. I'm learning to tame that voice. And though it's a work in progress, there are times when that voice calms down. That voice takes a breath. Retrained, unable to ignore or minimize my achievements, it smiles, and says, "good job."

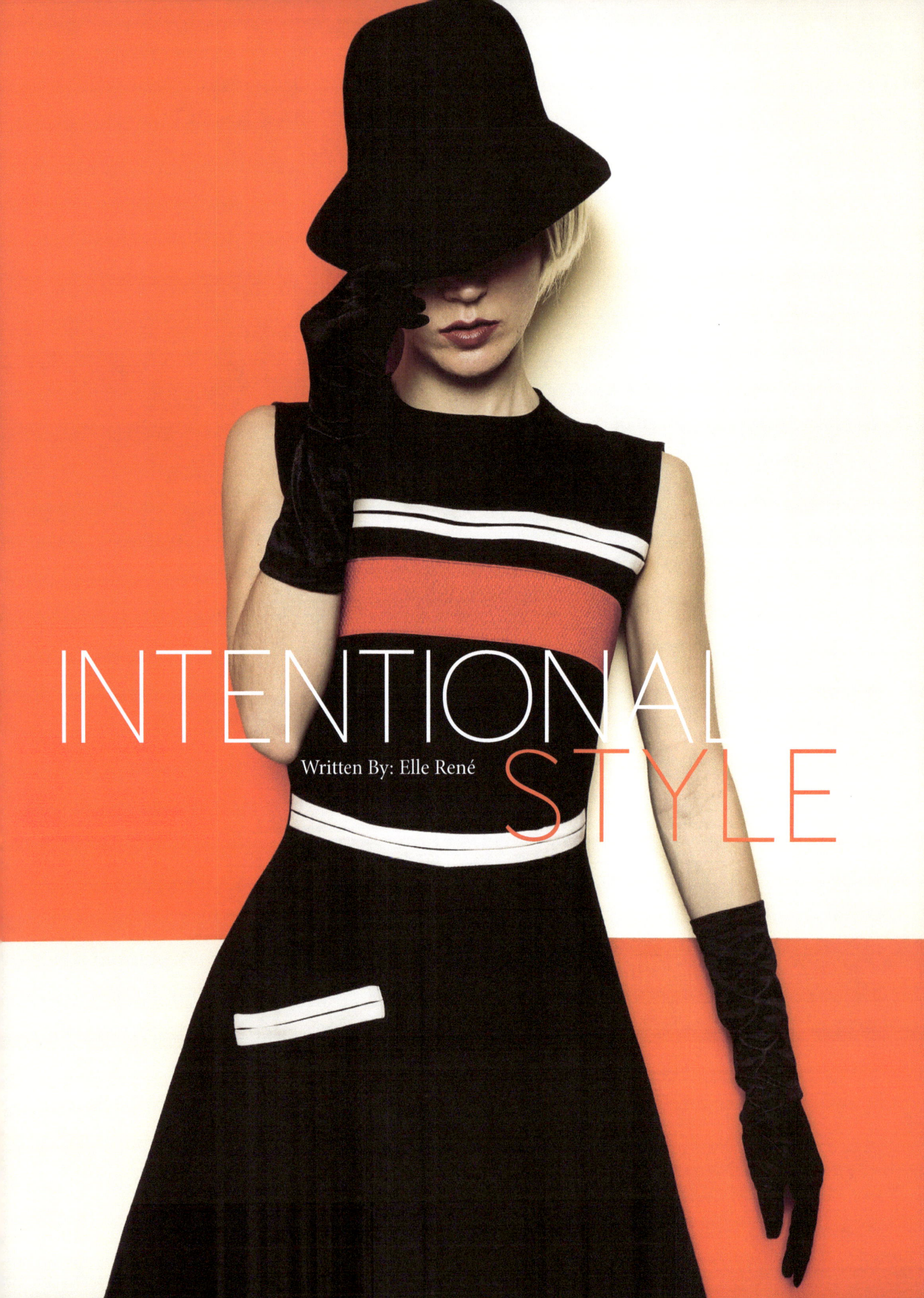

INTENTIONAL STYLE

Written By: Elle René

Fashion is what you buy. Style is how you wear it. Expressing yourself through style is probably more nerve-wracking than preparing a speech or for an interview. But if I could offer one piece of advice, it be not to let the thought of getting dressed scare you. In fact, you could get excited about what you were going to wear, if you knew what you should wear.

If you took some time and went through your closet, you would mostly like agree that every piece of clothing rather hanging up, folded up or buried in the pile became a part of wardrobe, or every piece of jewelry you own, because it had a purpose. You intended to wear it to work, church, school, date night, for an interview or during your much needed "me" time. Being intentional about the choices you make are not only relevant in the other areas of your life, but also when it comes to your style.

Here are three ways the woman pharmacist can present themselves with *intentional style*:

STYLE & HUE.

Colors have a simple yet powerful ability to set the "feel". With every room you walk into, you have the opportunity to be the thermostat and not the thermometer, meaning you set the tone instead of adapting to what already exists. When selecting the hue you want to wear, be intentional to ensure it aligns with your message and reflects your style. Hues have been known to the influence someone's perception. For example, red grabs attention, blue promotes trust and loyalty, while brown shows dependability and honesty. Choose wisely…choose style.

STYLE & STRUCTURED.

As a woman constantly on the go, you may find it tempting to carry not only things you need, but everything you think you will need. We have all had those "what if" and "I should have brought" moments when heading to a meeting or work. Even in those moments, stay structured.

Carry a purse, briefcase or portfolio, that is structured and sturdy. Avoid bling, tassels and other distracting applications. You never know who is watching.

STYLE & SMILE.

Flash your million-dollar smile. They say a smile is worth a thousand words, so without ever saying one word, believe it or not, your smile speaks volumes. Investing in teeth whitening products is another way to enhance your image. Discolored teeth can cheapen your look, so level up and brighten up your smile. Before you know it you will find yourself intentionally smiling to match your intentional style.

About the Author

Elle Renée is personal image consultant. Founder of Hoosier Stylist & Image Consultant, Elle Renée helps women and men build wardrobes that reflect their ambition, brilliance and confidence in style. Connect with Elle Renée @hoosierstylist on FB and IG.

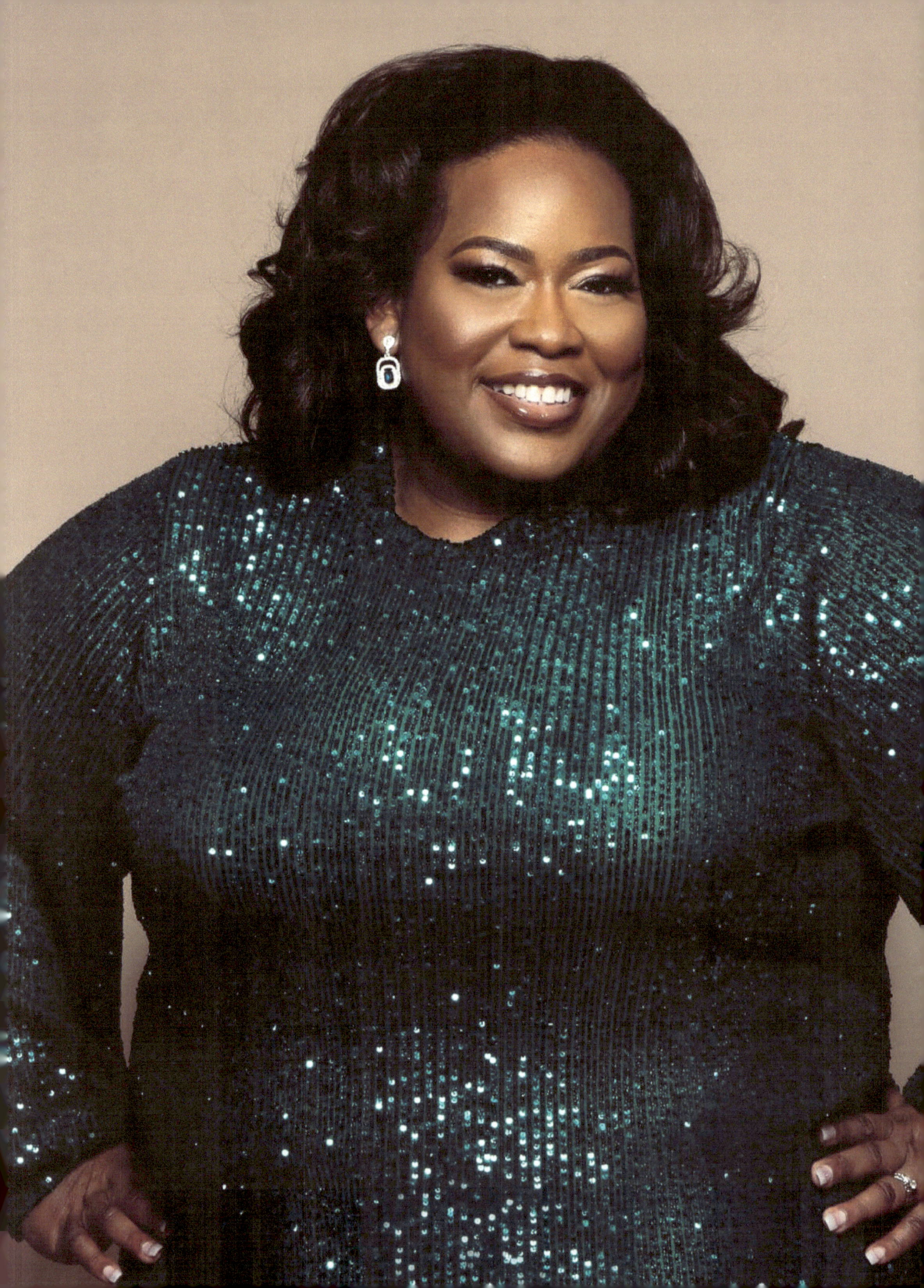

WHERE ARE THEY NOW

Dr. Leslie Hodge

Start. Go. Do.

INDIANAPOLIS | PHARMACY SCHOOL: **PURDUE UNIVERSITY** | DEGREES: **PHARMD** |
PREVIOUS CAREER: **RETAIL PHARMACY MANAGER, CONSULTANT PHARMACIST AND PERSONAL STYLIST & IMAGE CONSULTANT** |
NOW CAREER: **ADJUNCT PROFESSOR, FOUNDER OF EMERGE LEARNING INSTITUTE PHARMACY TECHNICIAN TRAINING AND CERTIFICATION PROGRAM, CONSULTANT PHARMACIST AND PERSONAL STYLIST & IMAGE CONSULTANT**

Tell us more of your story...So what happened next?.

I had the nudge to leave retail pharmacy for at least the last three to five years. No, nothing was wrong, I just knew there was more for me to do.

The fear of being somewhere longer than I was supposed to be outweighed the fear of the disrupting or interrupting what had been consistent for the past 17 years - being a pharmacist and pharmacy manager.

My time to say YES to me, the unknown, the interruption and to the world of opportunities finally revealed itself in July 2022.

There is a saying that if you want to make God laugh, tell Him your plans. Well, my plan was to take at least the following three months off to rest, travel and do the things I had missed out on over the years due to my work schedule. Well, that quickly changed when 9 days after my last day l was sitting in a panel interview for an adjunct professor position for a dual credit early college high school program. Three months of resting and traveling became three weeks because the first day of school was during the last week of July.

As I look back over the past few years, I rejoice, celebrate and thank God daily for waiting on me to say yes to His plan, His will and His timing for my life, because truth be told, I thought I was waiting on Him.

I never knew what was on the other side of my yes, but I am eternally grateful for the countless opportunities that have come my way.

What section of the PharmaSis Magazine were you originally featured?

Fall 2019

How were you featured in the magazine?

Featured Pharmacist

What's new since you last appeared in PharmaSis Magazine?

Since my appearance in the premier issue of PharmaSis Magazine I left retail pharmacy and

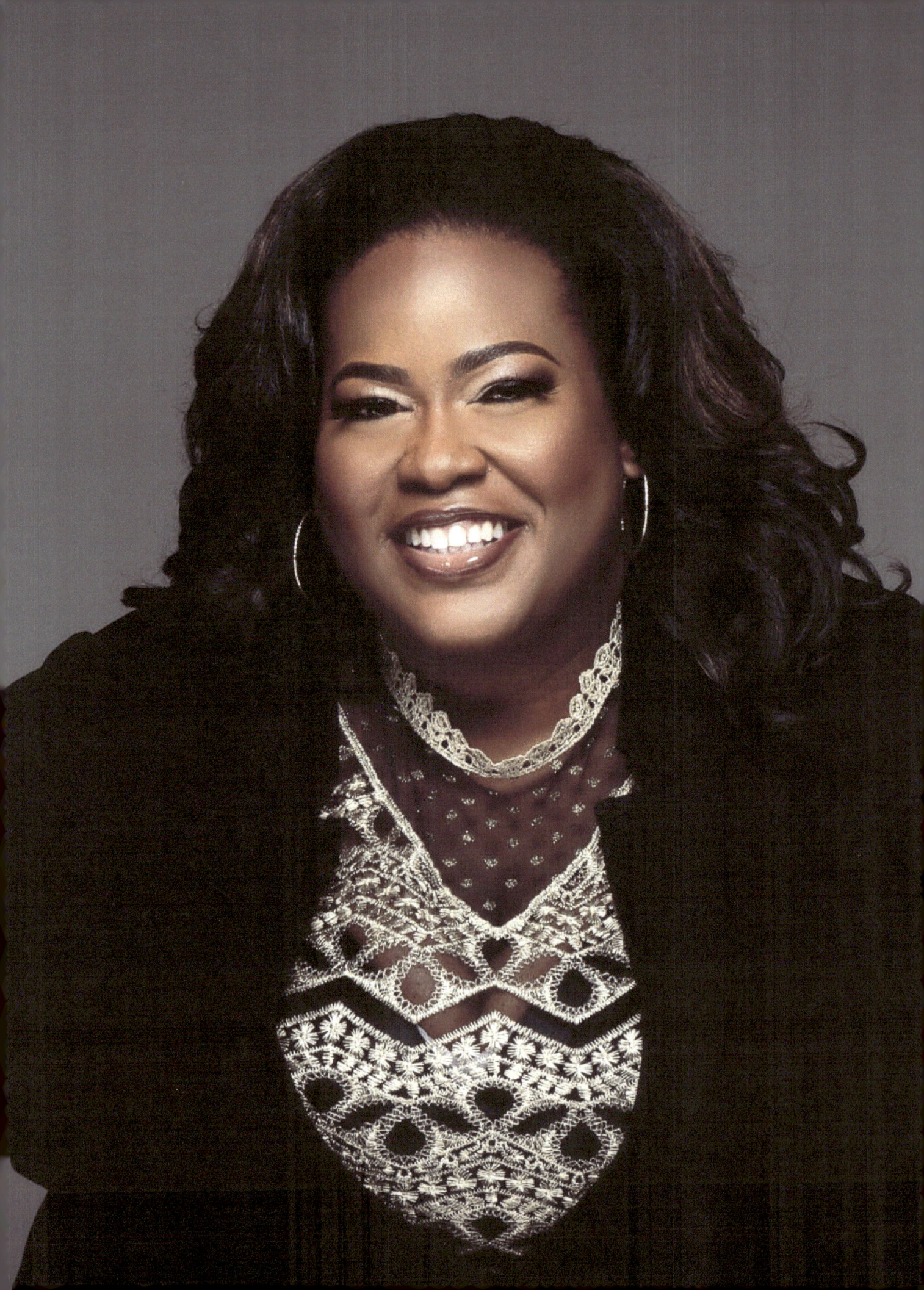

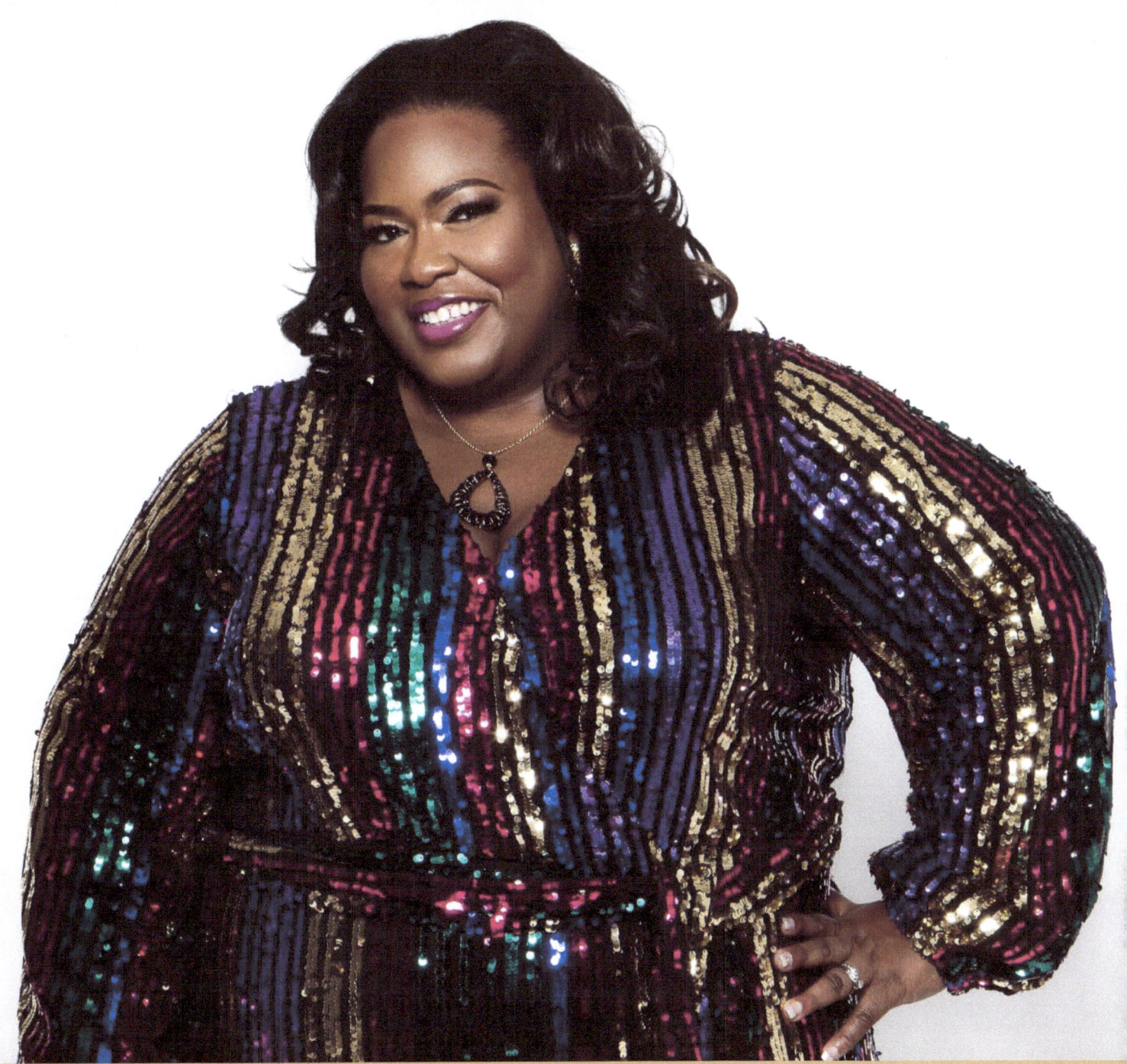

now teach and train the next generation of healthcare providers through an adjunct professor position with a dual credit early college high school program and through Emerge Learning Institute, LLC - an institute I founded that offers a pharmacy technician training and certification program. Scripts & Beyond, LLC continues to provide medication consultation services and impact communities through our health education programs. Lastly, but certainly not least, I continue to take my passion for fashion to the heights through Hoosier Stylist and Image Consultant, where I help female entrepreneurs, experts and executives reflect their ambition, brilliance and confidence in style.

Any advice for Women in Pharmacy that you would like to share:
Start. Go. Do. Be unapologetically YOU. Extend yourself and others grace.

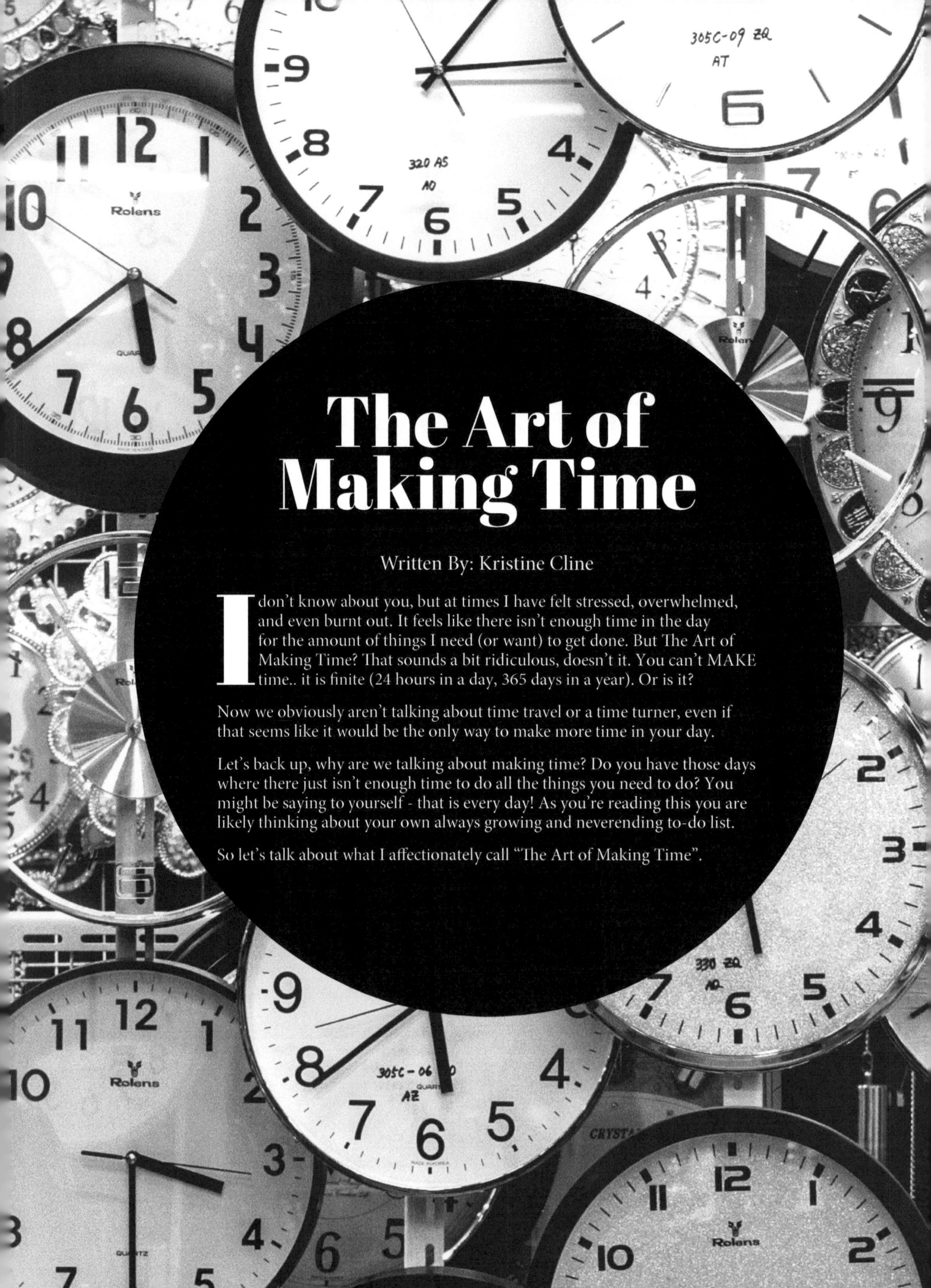

The Art of Making Time

Written By: Kristine Cline

I don't know about you, but at times I have felt stressed, overwhelmed, and even burnt out. It feels like there isn't enough time in the day for the amount of things I need (or want) to get done. But The Art of Making Time? That sounds a bit ridiculous, doesn't it. You can't MAKE time.. it is finite (24 hours in a day, 365 days in a year). Or is it?

Now we obviously aren't talking about time travel or a time turner, even if that seems like it would be the only way to make more time in your day.

Let's back up, why are we talking about making time? Do you have those days where there just isn't enough time to do all the things you need to do? You might be saying to yourself - that is every day! As you're reading this you are likely thinking about your own always growing and neverending to-do list.

So let's talk about what I affectionately call "The Art of Making Time".

1. **Prioritize** - What NEEDS to get done today? What are your goals? Think about this before you write down or look at your to-do list.

2. **Write it down** - It can be tempting to make the list first, but don't let the "what" cloud the "why". Brain dump, word vomit, put everything that needs to happen that is taking up your cognitive energy and write it all down.

3. **Take a break** - Whew! That was a lot of work. Treat yo' self! Go for a stroll, eat lunch, kick your feet up and watch that show you've wanted to catch up on.

4. **Be realistic** - Have you read Stephen Covey's "The 7 Habits of Highly Effective People"? One of my favorite parts of the book is the concept of the 4 quadrants:

Urgent and Important	**Not Urgent but Important**
Urgent but Not Important	**Neither Urgent nor Important**

So often we treat everything has priority #1 - urgent and important. This can leave us feeling like all we do is put out fire after fire. That is exhausting! But what about all of the other important things in our lives? How do we go from reactive to proactive? (That's a million dollar question!)

We tend to address urgent things first, regardless of importance. Obviously there will be things that come up that are both urgent and important, but try to make a conscious effort to focus your energy and time on things that are IMPORTANT. Consider arranging your to-do list in this manner to help you prioritize.

5. **Decision time** - the 5 D's (not of dodgeball, but of making time!)

    Delete - lots of things on our mental radar (or in our inbox) can just be deleted. Do I really NEED to do this? Prioritizing your list using the 4 quadrants can help with this

    Do - I like to use the "5 minute rule". If there are things that will take me less than 5 minutes, I do those first to get the feeling of momentum. And who doesn't like crossing lots of things off the list quickly?

    Delegate - this one is hard. Are there things on your personal list that can be delegated to a partner? Or things on your work list you are holding on to that a coworker can/should do? Evaluate which things do YOU need to be the one to do?

    Defer - this is another place where prioritizing using the 4 quadrants helps. Which things are not urgent or important (that you didn't already delete) can be deferred to later?

    Dance - you did it! Getting used to prioritizing and using the 5 D's can feel like a lot of work at first. It does get easier with practice. In the meantime, dance and celebrate your hard work and your investment in yourself.

Sounds easy peasy, right? NO!! The Art of Making Time is HARD WORK. Give yourself grace as you adjust to this new process of prioritizing your tasks. Every little steps gets you closer to more time for you and your loved ones.

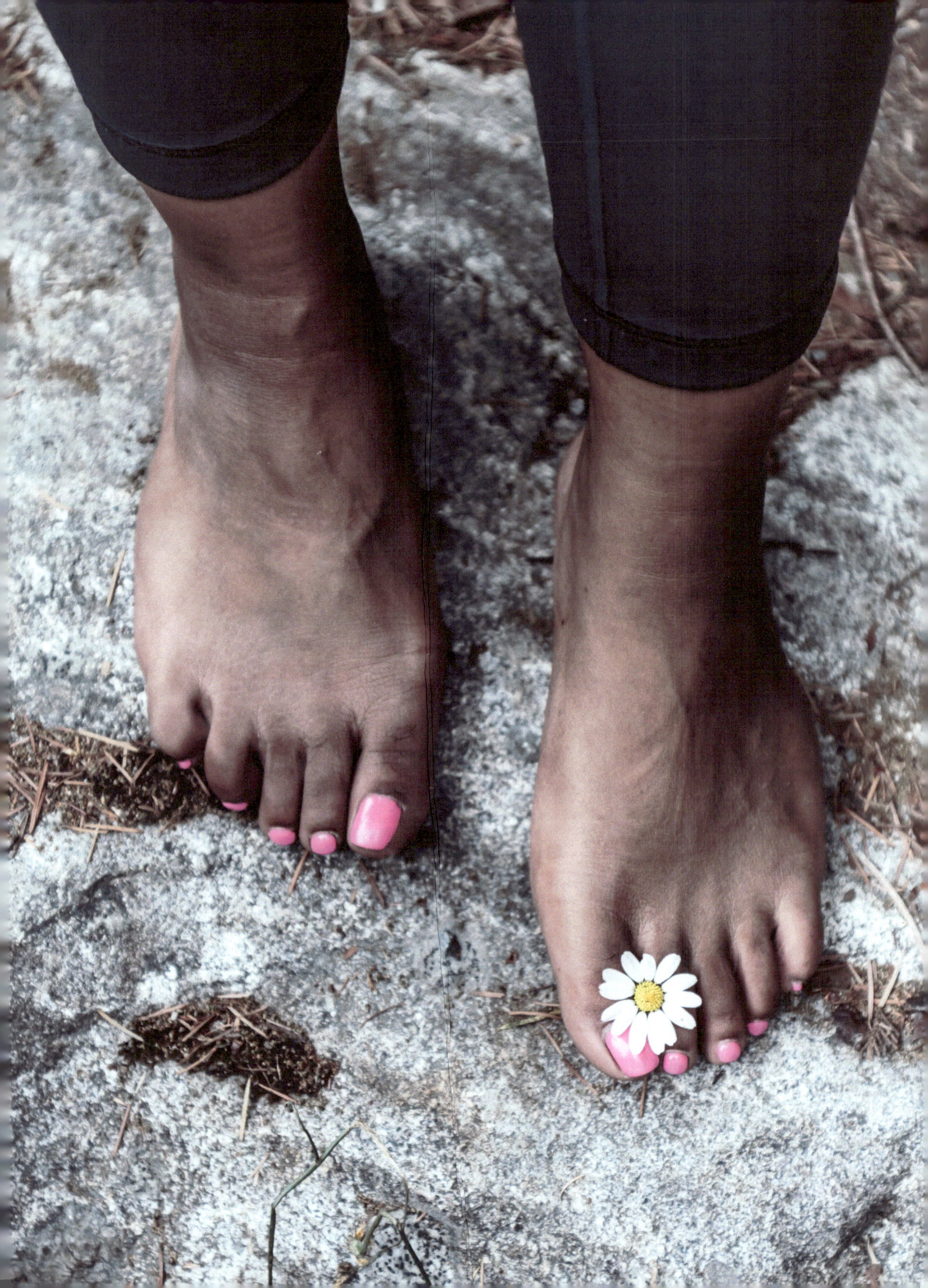

I DARE YOU TO BARE YOUR SOLES

Written By: Dr. Gilda M. Jefferson

I've always hated wearing shoes, especially as a child! Nothing makes my heart more content than to bare my feet and absorb Mother Earth's free-flowing energy.

Barefoot and free, playing and grounding for health and vitality!

Grounding, also known as Earthing, is an energetic phenomenon that occurs when bare skin comes in direct contact with Mother Earth. Per thejoywithin.org, it is defined as the mental, emotional, and spiritual process of rooting your consciousness back into connection with the earth. Love it!

Did you know being indoors and wearing rubber-soled shoes every time you leave home disconnects you from the earth's electricity? That's correct, modern life can negatively impact your body.

Technology is full of ions that pollute your body; they are positive and have "dirty energy". Natural dirt, on the contrary, is enriched with much-needed negative ions that neutralize toxins - your body craves daily doses. Exposing your body to more positive than negative ions can wreak havoc on your health.

The solution? Become a Barefoot PharmD!

Softly walk barefoot on Mother Earth daily. When the soles of your feet make contact, the magic begins. Harmful positive ions neutralize, and your energetic body becomes balanced.

Life is all about balance. As an earthly being, you are to live and commune with other earthly beings - nature is your vital life source. Living with nature, vitality, and prosperity are signs of a well-balanced life.

Not convinced grounding is for you? Let's give it a try!

Kick your shoes off…stand quietly or walk slowly in the dirt/grass for 8 -11 minutes.

What are your soles feeling? is the dirt/grass cool? moist? hard? soft? Any rocks?

Note: There is no pain in this process - there are only sensations that will soon pass.

Focus on your breathing - slowly inhale and exhale through your nose.

For the duration, silently repeat "All I am (inhaling), is my breath (exhaling)"

Continue breathing and repeating the mantra; now focus energy on your heart.

Eventually, its beat will sync to the rhythm of Mother Earth.

Imagine… Your soles to soul Recalibration!

Now… How do you feel?

Besides Mother Earth missing connection with you, here are a few more motivational benefits of grounding:

- strengthens immune system
- improves cognitive and physical function
- decreases pain, muscle tension, and stress
- decreases affinity for anxiety and depression
- Improves sleep quality, vitality, and overall health

I dare you to bare Your soles and connect with Mother Earth daily!

What's the BEST that could happen!?

If you have any questions, do not hesitate to contact me.

Your Barefoot PharmaSis

Dr.Gilda ~ TheWriteClinician

Dr. Gilda M. Jefferson, founder of TheWriteClinician, LLC

A featured pharmacist and contributing author to PharmaSis Magazine

Contact: https://bit.ly/GildaJefferson

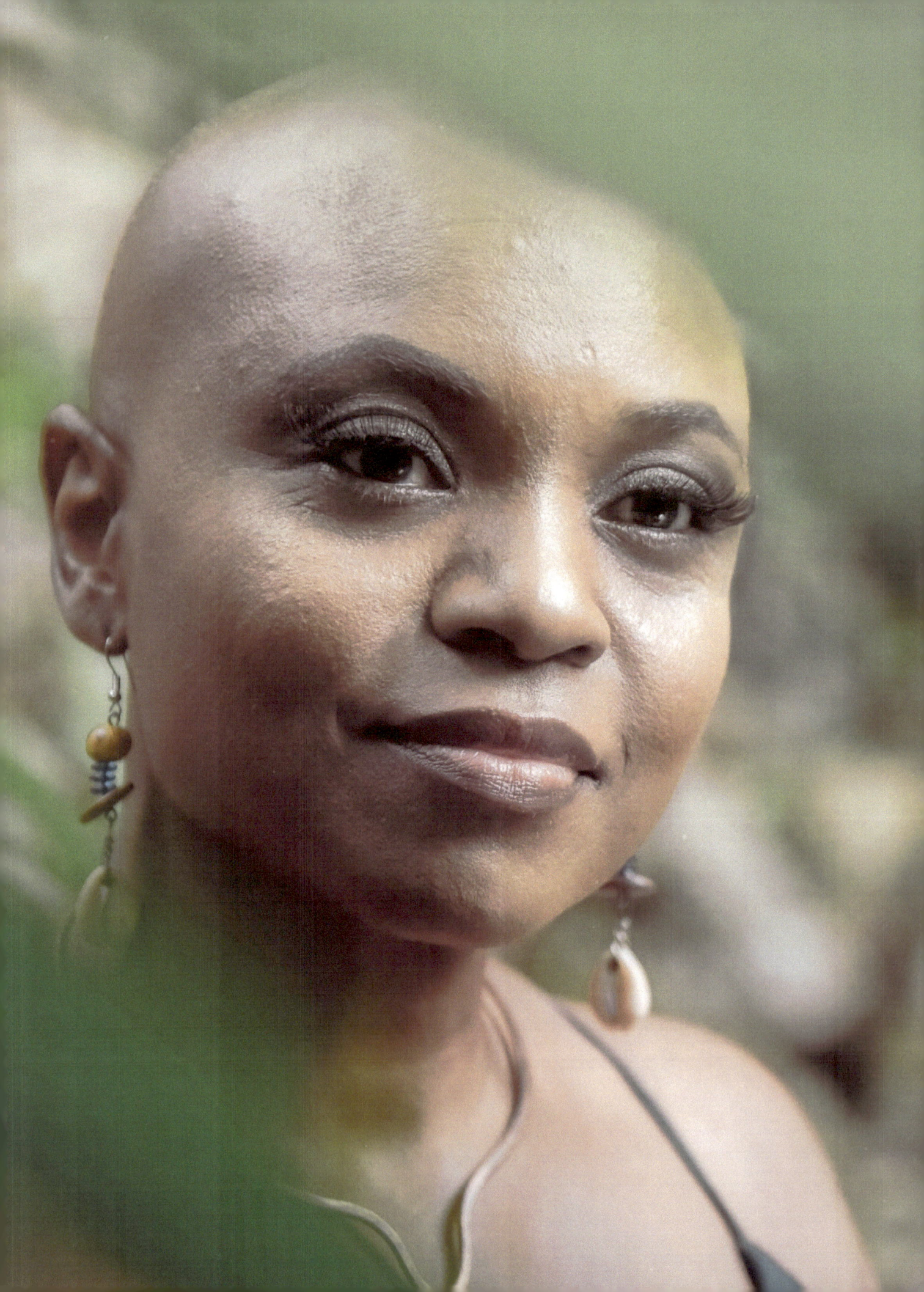

AUTHOR SPOTLIGHT

DR. GILDA M. JEFFERSON
From Foster Care to Freedom: My Journey to Radical Self-Love and Authenticity

Tell us a little about yourself!

Growing up in California's foster care system, my childhood was a cesspool of abuse and neglect. Yet, I persevered!

College to adulting was interesting and unfulfilling...

Leaving spare time to collect a few more titles (US Army veteran, Dr. of Pharmacy, health coach, functional medicine practitioner, naturopath, etc) along the way.

Somewhere, somehow I lost me...

Correction, imposter syndrome triggered a recollection of who I truly was.

So, off I went on a remembrance quest.

Divinely guided to ancient lands, I've been honored to train with traditional medicine women and men. And due to fear/judgment of others, and my own limiting beliefs I've not lived My Truth nor fully embraced Me.

Today I embrace ALL parts of Me... free to flow and grow ~

I've released ALL toxicity accumulated during my time in the Rx profession.

Most importantly, I forgive Self for allowing and staying past the expiration dates.

As diagnoses of stress-induced auto-immune diseases such as Lupus and Mixed-connected tissue disease and more... Were not worthy of Me.

Due to my inability adequately verbalize my pain, or burden another, my fur baby and I left the US...After selling my house and giving away 90% of my worldly possessions.

Liberation!!

Until the real work began... Complete Dissection of My Beingness.

With my tattered mind, body, and essence strewn across the lab's linoleum steel countertop...

I was Divinely guided on the path of Radical Self-love. And taught how to gingerly collect my parts, integrate and heal them holistically.

Though the prognosis was bleak, the outcome has been magical.

Psst! No hair was lost in this experiment, I am bald by choice.

Describe your passion and why it's important.

I am passionate about LIFE and being authentic! Our interactions with all creatures should come from a place of empathy and compassion and not one of an opportunist -- as we are all important.

What do you want women in pharmacy to take away from your expertise shared in your articles

I desire women in pharmacy to consider alternative healing modalities, for themselves and others. Additionally, we are all here for a purpose beyond work; don't be afraid to follow your intuition to live your authentic truth.

Tell us a fun fact about yourself!

My name means Golden... And I am an Alkhemist

Saltwater is my sanctuary where remoras love to hitch a ride when I dive.

Facebook: gilda.jeffersun/

IG: @gj.apothecary

X: web3_scribe

Website: thewriteclinician.com

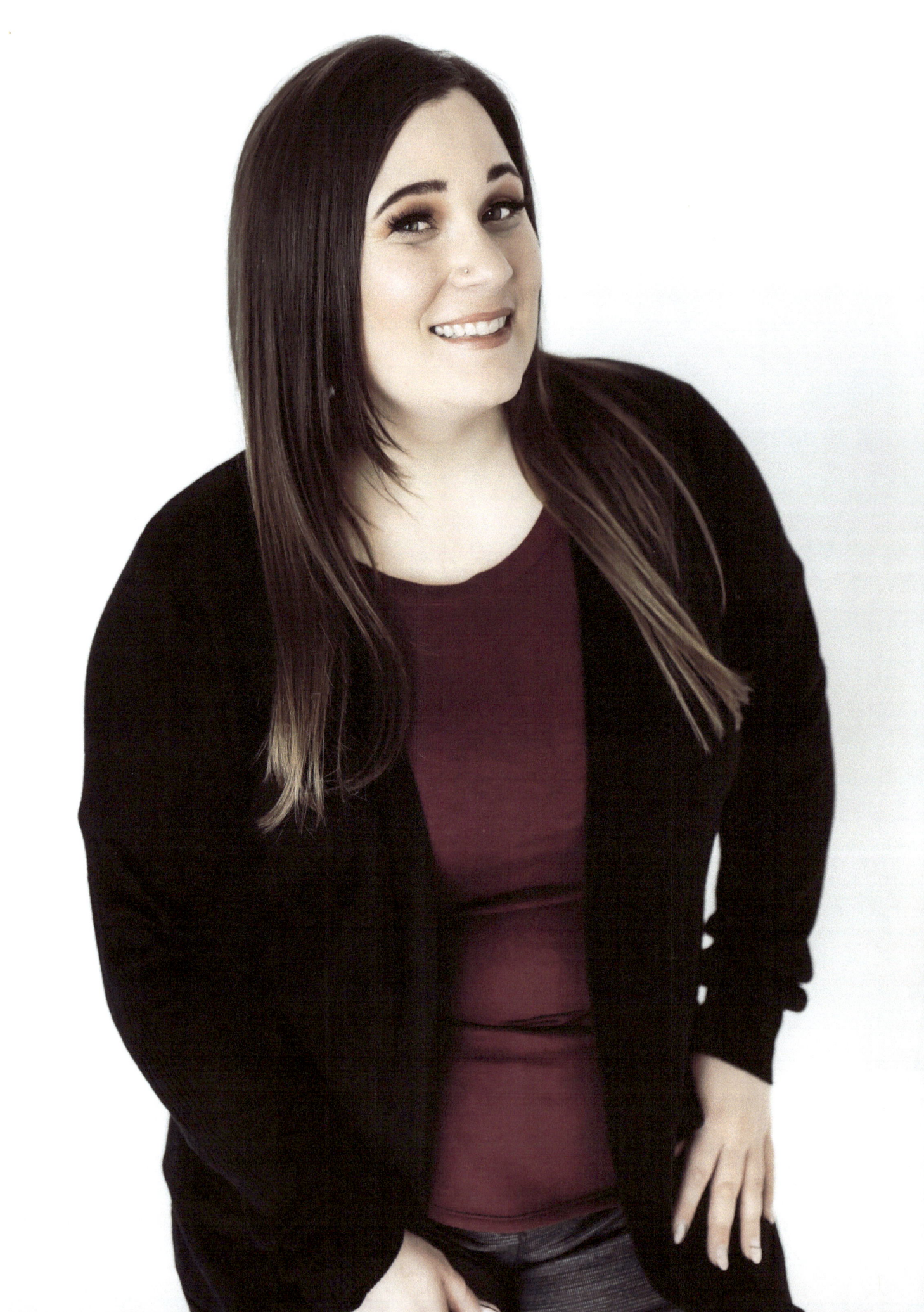

APPRENTICESHIP CONSULTING PHARMACY
COMPOUNDING SERVICES

Whitney Jo Hummel

Leading with Compassion

FORT MYERS, FL | PHARMACY SCHOOL: **SOUTH FLORIDA STATE COLLEGE** | DEGREES: **BA.A.S. AT SOUTH FLORIDA STATE COLLEGE, PRACTICAL NURSING CERTIFICATE AT SOUTH FLORIDA STATE COLLEGE, YOGA INSTRUCTOR CERTIFICATION,** | PREVIOUS CAREER: **PHARMACY OPERATIONS COORDINATOR** | NOW CAREER : **APPRENTICESHIP CONSULTING PHARMACY COMPOUNDING SERVICES**

Tell your story...how did you get here?

I had a difficult childhood and those that know my story are often astounded by how far I have come. I grew up in a small rural town environment where both of my parents had severe addiction problems that would periodically result in legal problems. As a result, I was often negatively judged, while growing up, because of my parent's problems. I often thought that if I had grown up in a bigger city there would not have been as much attention on my family. In small towns, everyone seems to know everyone else's business, especially in circumstances like my family's. I was labeled as a child from an unfit home. Even some teachers had cast these judgments on me before I was able to prove myself in the classroom. Many of my classmates were forewarned, by their parents, to not associate with me. Another obstacle for me was being diagnosed with a learning disability at four years old that made it difficult to speak. This made it very hard to speak up for myself, even though on the inside I knew what I wanted to say.

No one knew that my father chastised me constantly. I was pressured by him to not talk because he did not want me to tell teachers what was happening at home. I believe this was not recognized by others for the following reasons. First, teachers and psychologists never looked too deeply because I came from a broken home. Secondly, since I was labeled as having a "learning disability". I had an older brother who was highly intelligent and well-liked at school. My father told my brother that if the teachers ever questioned him about things I said that he was supposed to tell them I had many issues and did not know what I was talking about. Since my older brother was well-respected, many teachers believed anything he said. As a result, I felt constrained and judged by others at school. Interestingly, my mother grew up in the same small town as I did and was known as mischievous and a party girl. Many people in the town knew this about her and assumed I was the same way which is the furthest from the truth. I often thought about how I could escape this situation.

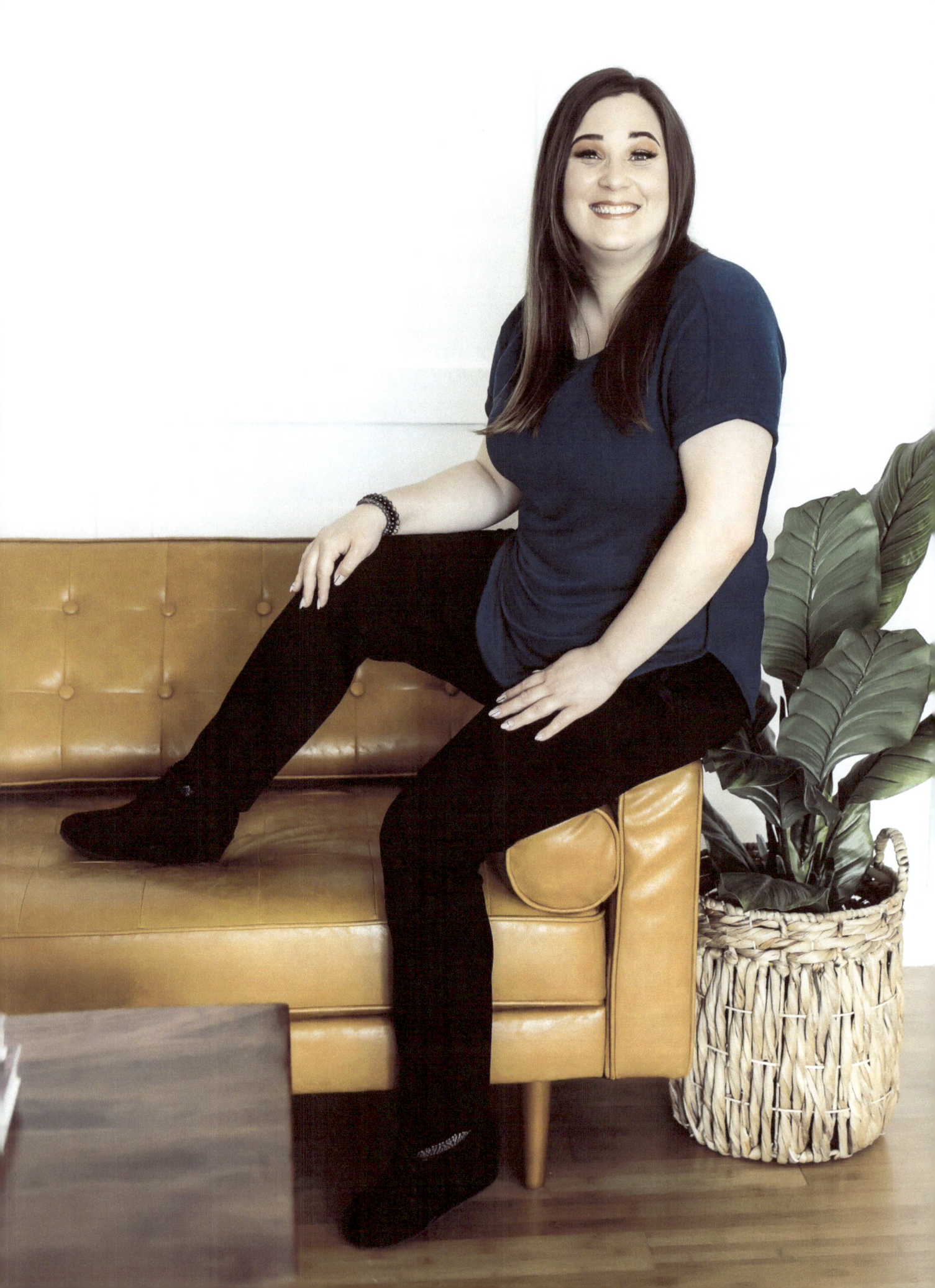

As a result of my tough start in the world, my elementary school years were not very memorable. I was not able to speak my thoughts clearly until I was in 4th grade, which prevented me from expressing my feelings for a very long time. I felt different from other children and was trapped in myself without the ability to express myself. However, I knew I was smart, had a strong will, and just wanted a chance to prove myself to others. Since I was one of the younger students in my class and had a very emotional time in elementary school, which was perceived as a learning disability, I was given a chance to repeat the 5th grade. I decided that I would take this opportunity to create a blank slate for myself with new peers. I really pushed myself that year earning straight A's and even being awarded the presidential physical fitness award. Repeating 5th grade was one of the best decisions to begin to build my self-confidence. For the first time in 10 years, I could shine a little and show my true colors!

This doesn't mean my life was easy after this because I was still haunted by my past until I graduated high school because of the small-town agenda. I did not let this stop me. By this time, it began to fuel my ambition, drive, and energy to focus on creating a better life. I always believed that no one knew me better than myself. I was not going to let others define me or define my future. Some of the worst pains can be channeled to make someone a better, stronger, and more powerful person. I think this is why God says not to judge others. Almost no one knew about my situation at home or how I had to bear torment in my younger years. Many people judged my situation instead of understanding it and me. It goes to show that you never know anyone's true story. As painful as this experience was, it has helped develop my character and define me as a person. I always try to understand where people are coming from and tell myself there is always more than what you see or hear. It should never be our place to judge others but help people to the best of our abilities.

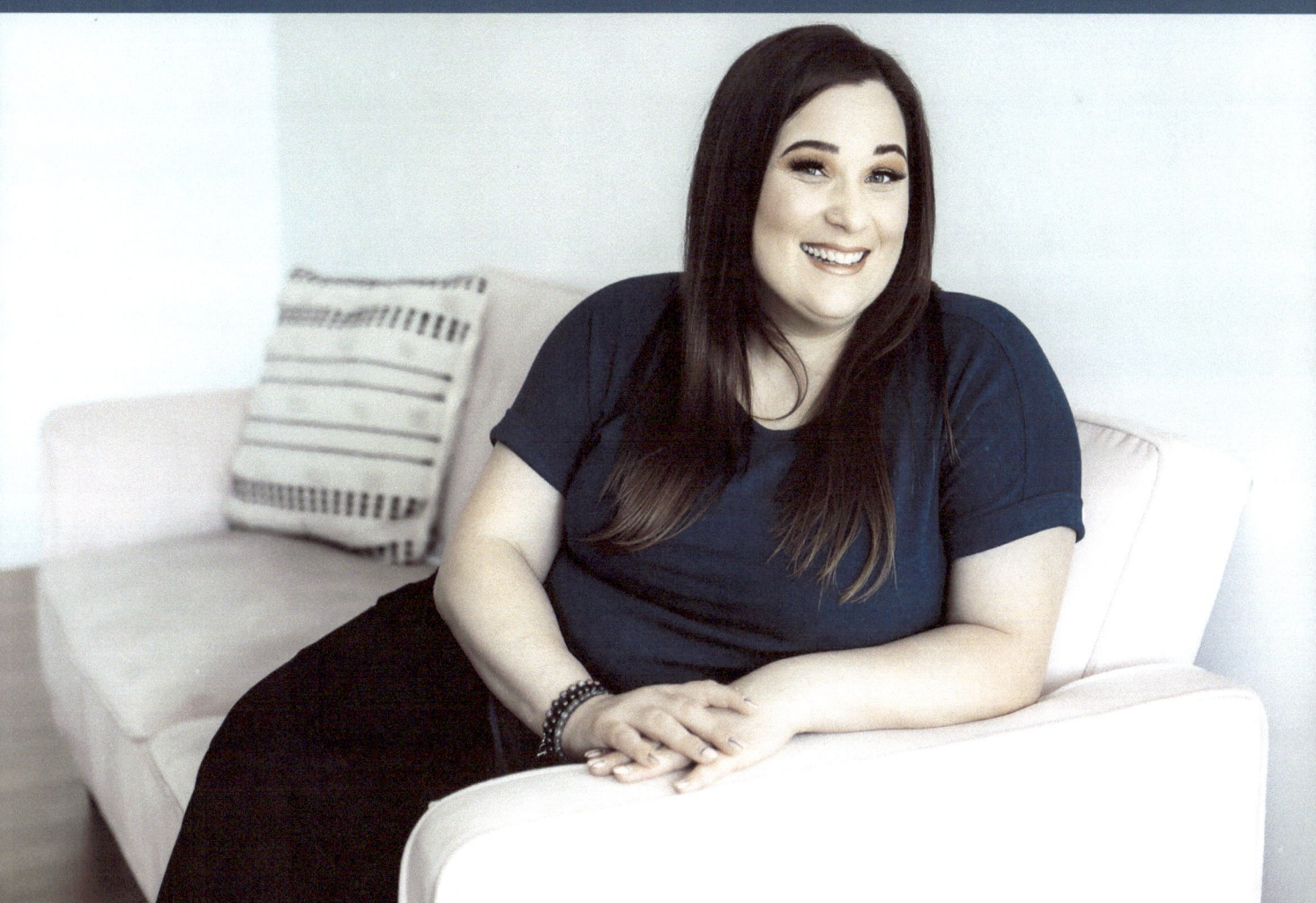

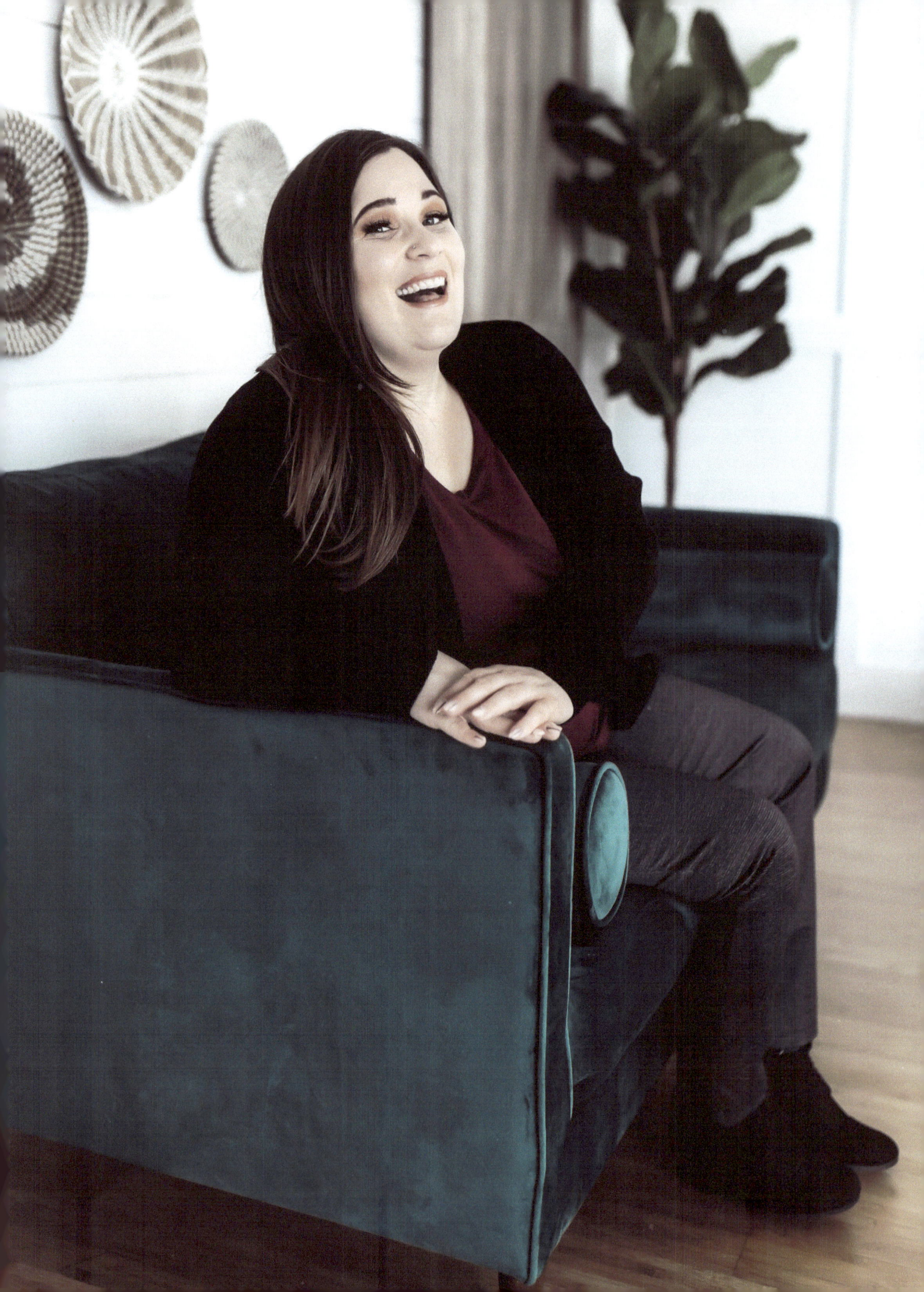

Describe what you are building/have built (your business; your career)

I continue to build my certifications in different areas. A primary interest of mine is vegan cooking, yoga instructing, and a holistic lifestyle. I have an A.A.S. degree since 2011, but I plan to further my education.

What's been your biggest lesson you have learned along your journey?

Setting healthy boundaries for yourself so others will respect you. This also means you must have respect for yourself.

How do you respond to fear?

I try to rationalize the fear. I never try to let fear drive me.

What does it mean to be considered a leader in your profession and industry?

A leader, to me, is someone who holds true to their word, someone who follows through and is willing to learn and understand others. We primarily work with patients' lives, so I think having compassion for our patients and colleagues in the field is vital.

At this time, pharmacists are being challenged to think out of the box more than ever. What advice do you have for the pharmacist who is wondering how to do that?

First, you must know where you want to focus in the pharmacy world. What does this look like for you? After envisioning this dream, start to make small steps to achieve that goal. Once you hit the marks on the small goals, keep making new goals. Each time making the goal size a little bit bigger. Make connections with people that have achieved your dream. Learning from others is always the best approach!

Who do you look up to or model yourself after (personal or professional)?

The biggest role models in my life are those who are the closest to me, including my husband, family, and friends. I firmly believe in the adage that "we are who we walk with" and I am grateful to be surrounded by those who consistently challenge me, shower me with love, show me lifelong lessons, and be my rock of support.

What message would you share with other colleagues in pharmacy?

Follow your intuition on situations. If something doesn't feel right, it probably isn't.

What characteristics do you feel you have had to grow or display most during your journey?

Reminding myself that we all are on different paths in life. Instead of judging others, we should to understand what is life to be in that individuals shoes. Having deeper compassion for others.

What's next for you and/or your business?

To be determined. Sometimes pausing your life always allows you to see the bigger picture. It is okay to pause! We live in a busy culture, but resting and reflecting when needed are okay and can really help. I feel we all need this reminder sometimes in life.

Where can we find you to further connect?

https://www.linkedin.com/in/whitneyjohummel/

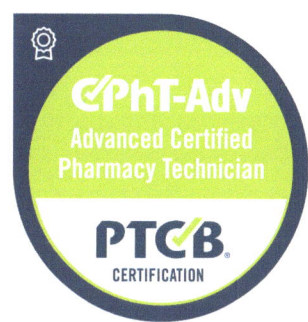
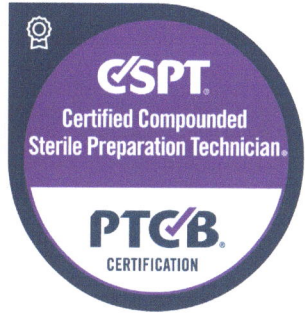

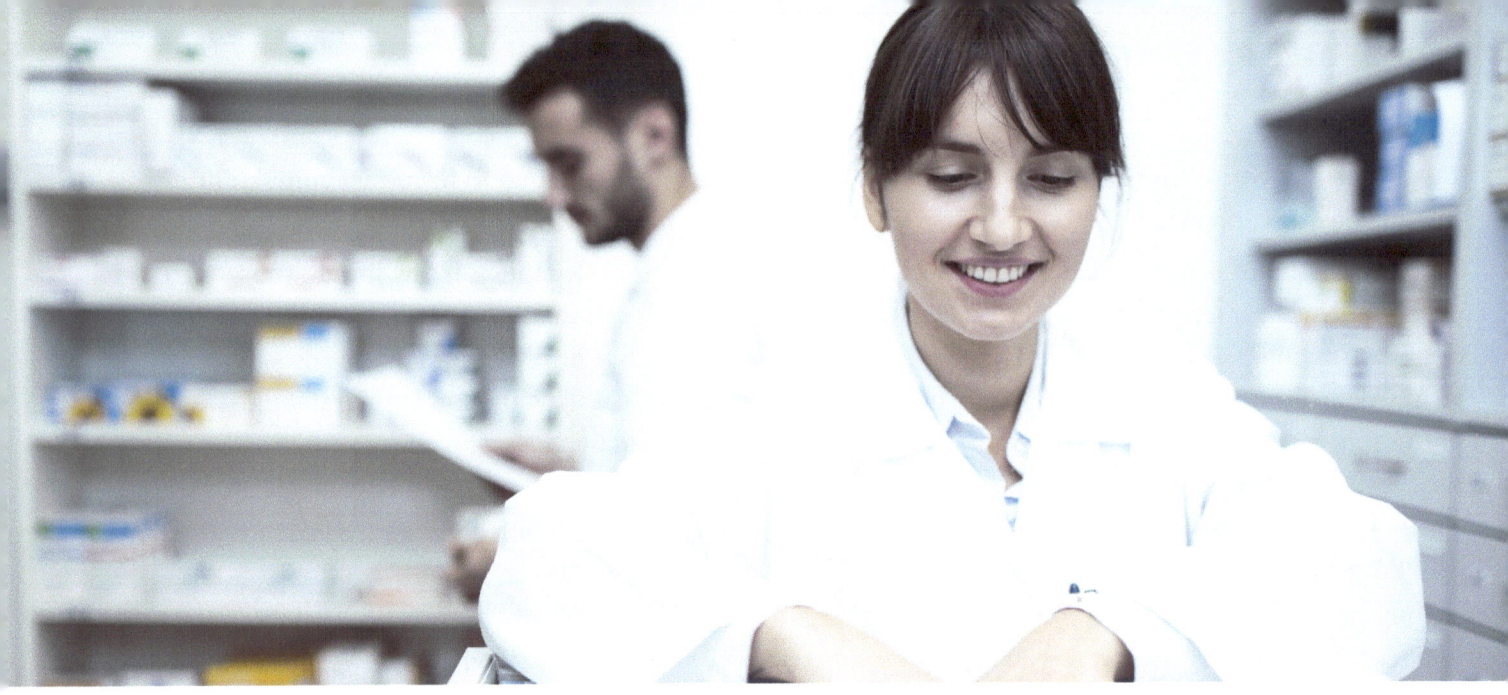

A Special Message to Pharmacy Technicians

Written By: Whitney Jo Hummel

The strain caused by the pandemic has intensified the importance of pharmacy technicians in the workplace. Technicians, among other medical professionals, were worked very hard throughout this crisis, but do not always receive the recognition they deserve. During this pandemic, the importance and value of pharmacy technicians were truly recognized by health professionals, as well as customers. Pharmacy technicians were likely selling themselves short for a long time, and now is an opportunity to recognize our worth and what we bring to the table.

Organizations like the Pharmacy Technician Certification Board (PTCB) and the National Pharmacy Technician Association (NPTA) offer certifications for technician advancement. These certifications can help you to become more knowledgeable in the many facets of pharmacy, as well as showing ambition in your career. Attaining these certifications shows (tangibly) that you have attained knowledge in a particular area which can be key to elevating yourself in this field. Other examples of how to elevate yourself is to create a LinkedIn page, get involved in a pharmacy association, write pharmacy-related articles, present webinars/ CEs, and learn non-pharmacy skillsets that can be applied in pharmacy settings. This can set you apart from other candidates for a position you may be seeking. Connections is probably what matters most! Building a solid reputation showing what you have to offer will lead to opportunities with diligence.

Likely the most important piece of advice I can give you, from my technician experience, is to not stay at a place that hired you to do a set of tasks, but has you do something completely different, if you are not happy. Get to know your work setting, employees, and managers and see if it is a good fit for you. Do not gamble and waste your time hoping the situation will change. Try to gather as much information as possible before, evaluate the situation, and see if the new opportunity serves you. Time is precious. Ask as many questions as possible as you need to improve your satisfaction and assess the situation carefully. Do not settle for less. Visualize the life you desire and aim for that goal. Challenges will arise, but how we navigate and approach them will make our journey smoother.

www.ingramcontent.com/pod-product-compliance
Lightning Source LLC
Chambersburg PA
CBHW051218220526
45473CB00003B/1080